Advance Praise for
Food Truths from Farm to Table

"This book is for the 7 billion people who eat each day. Michele Payn highlights how family farms are fighting food waste, hunger, and other issues, and the solutions they're coming up with in fields across the world."
—**Danielle Nierenberg, *Food Tank***

"Smart grocery shopping and healthy eating shouldn't require a science degree. *Food Truths from Farm to Table* guides you through the grocery store and saves you time. If you are looking to shop and eat with less guilt, read this book. Michele's 25 food truths will give you the freedom to enjoy your food again."
—**Phil Lempert, The Supermarket Guru, former NBC News' *Today Show* Food Trends Editor, author, and speaker**

"This is an important topic whether you are an academic, dietitian or consumer. Michele Payn's 25 food truths are grounded in science and she offers an unheard voice in the debate around food, nutrition and health. If you want to give yourself permission to be smart about food, read *Food Truths from Farm to Table* today."
—**Sonya Meyer, PhD, Director, Margaret Ritchie School of Family & Consumer Sciences, University of Idaho**

"Buy, prepare and serve healthy, affordable food with confidence after reading *Food Truths from Farm to Table: 25 Surprising Ways to Shop & Eat without Guilt*. This book is must-read for anyone interested in food, nutrition and health!"
—**Elizabeth Pivonka, PhD, RD, President & CEO of Produce for Better Health Foundation**

"In *Food Truths from Farm to Table*, Michele Payn cuts through the incredible noise that surrounds our food choices to provide clear, insightful answers to some of the most common questions about food. Organized in a creative way, she provides a highly informative 'guide book' to the grocery store, bringing both current research and insights from those who produce our food to unpack some of the most vexing questions and widespread myths about food. This candid and common-sense book will help you be a much more informed consumer and take the shame out of the food choices you make."
—**Jay Akridge, PhD, Glenn W. Sample Dean of Agriculture, Purdue University**

"Understanding the 'real story' about food is a critical issue for every health professional, parent, chef, and essentially anyone buying food. You will find answers to your most challenging questions around nutrition and health in *Food Truths from Farm to Table*—and learn to enjoy, not fear food."

—**Marianne Edge Smith, MS, RD, LD, FADA, FAND,**
Past President of Academy of Nutrition & Dietetics;
President, MSE & Associates, and farm owner

"As a dietitian for a grocery store chain, I know this book will not only help answer questions our customers have about the food they see on our shelves but also be a valuable resource to other supermarket dietitians throughout the country. Michele Payn gives practical insight to address myths around food, nutrition, and health. Read *Food Truths from Farm to Table* if you want to bring clarity to your food experience, based on science and real-life experience."

—**Leah McGrath, RDN, LDN**

"*Food Truths from Farm to Table* provides a transparent window into modern-day agriculture so you can better know the people and practices behind your food. Michele Payn has a unique ability to connect the values of farming and good buyers through story and science."

—**Charlie Arnot, CEO, Center for Food Integrity**

"Everyone can benefit from a clearer understanding of why farmers and ranchers produce food the way they do. Michele Payn takes readers inside farms and ranches to answer questions about the food issues on consumers' minds. *Food Truths from Farm to Table* provides a much-needed, well-rounded and accurate perspective on today's farming and ranching."

—**Zippy Duvall, President, American Farm Bureau Federation**

"This is an awesome book that provides usable information about food, farming, and nutrition. Michele Payn's insight is contrarian to the sensationalism of fashionable food, and will help you take the drama out of food choices. This book is an important read for every dietitian, grocery shopper, and anyone who wants to enjoy food."

—**Mary Lee Chin, MS, RD**

"It's time to celebrate and enjoy our abundant, wonderful food choices without angst, guilt, shame or fear. *Food Truths from Farm to Table* will help you be smart and comfortable about all food choices, while identifying marketing half-truths and misinformation that take the joy out of eating. Michele Payn connects farming, food, nutrition and health throughout this useful book."

—**Kim Galeaz, RDN, CD**

Food Truths
from
Farm to Table

Food Truths
from
Farm to Table

25 Surprising Ways
to Shop & Eat
without Guilt

Michele Payn

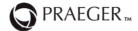 PRAEGER™

An Imprint of ABC-CLIO, LLC
Santa Barbara, California • Denver, Colorado

Library of Congress Cataloging-in-Publication Data

Names: Payn, Michele, author.
Title: Food truths from farm to table : 25 surprising ways to shop & eat
    without guilt / Michele Payn.
Description: Santa Barbara, California : Praeger, an imprint of ABC-CLIO,
    LLC, [2017] | Includes bibliographical references and index.
Identifiers: LCCN 2016052246 (print) | LCCN 2017000119 (ebook) |
    ISBN 9781440849978 (hard copy : alk. paper) | ISBN 9781440849985 (ebook)
Subjects: LCSH: Sustainable agriculture. | Food industry and trade. | Agriculture.
Classification: LCC S494.5.S86 P39 2017 (print) | LCC S494.5.S86 (ebook) |
    DDC 631.5—dc23
LC record available at https://lccn.loc.gov/2016052246

ISBN: 978-1-4408-4997-8
EISBN: 978-1-4408-4998-5

21 20 19 18 17   1 2 3 4 5

This book is also available as an eBook.

Praeger
An Imprint of ABC-CLIO, LLC

ABC-CLIO, LLC
130 Cremona Drive, P.O. Box 1911
Santa Barbara, California 93116-1911
www.abc-clio.com

This book is printed on acid-free paper ∞

Manufactured in the United States of America

To every person who has felt guilty or confused in the grocery store. May this book give you the permission to feel good about your family's food!

Contents

Acknowledgments

Gratitude to my daughter, who asked me daily how many words I had written and patiently listened to me pound away at the keyboard while you worked on chores, cattle, homework, and sports. I hope you are half as proud of my work as I am of you.

This book likely wouldn't have been completed without three people who challenged me nonstop. Thanks to Eliz, for the countless hours asking questions about claims in the grocery store; Jennie, my writing muse through volumes of research and spot-on edits; and Sam, my writing coach, who pushed me to translate the science through the stories of farmers and ranchers.

There are too many other people who helped to call out each individually. The 50+ farmers and ranchers, dietitians, scientists, veterinarians, and health professionals who so willingly shared their expertise—I appreciated our conversations. Likewise, a number of people at various organizations selflessly provided research and insight on these issues. More than 20 people served in an advisory community throughout the development of this book, providing invaluable guidance from all sides of the plate. Thank you to all of these folks serving the bigger picture of connecting farm to table. And to Elle for managing all the details.

In addition to their words of encouragement, gratitude to my personal friends for asking questions about their own food and bringing people together to discuss food myths. While your friendship is more important, the opportunity to share thoughts from your kitchen table is treasured. Your input kept me grounded in the highly emotional debate around food.

Audiences, from dietitians to ranchers, offered fodder over 15 years of speaking. The same can be said of my literary agent and online communities—sometimes just a question or simple comment provided perspective.

"A life without cause is a life without effect." This quote above my desk serves as a daily reminder of the cause of connecting farm and food. In short, thank you to each person who contributed to getting to the truth in food from the farm—your effect is found in these pages.

Introduction: Truth in Food

"Food is at the center of so many traditions. Food is essential to our bodies.
Food deserves to be celebrated, enjoyed, and shared.
The same could be said about the truth in food."

—Michele Payn

"I just want to have food that is good for my family. Why does it have to be so difficult?"

This was the question I kept hearing from a group of moms gathered around a long kitchen table on a cold January day.

I had asked them to get together to research how people felt going to the grocery store and to get their input on how food is grown. I wanted to learn from them so I could update my work to be relevant to people making food choices.

We talked about the agony of going to the grocery store. The guilt. The confusion.

"I don't have enough time to be researching all of this information. I just want to feed my family food I can trust. How can food be less confusing?"

The questions continued for two hours. "Why is finding the right food so confusing?" I asked.

As Ellen, a mom with four kids under the age of 11, said, "I don't know what to believe anymore. One year they tell us to avoid eggs, the next year we're supposed to only eat meat on certain days of the week and last week fruits were villains. I just want to be able to have food for my family that I know is healthy for them."

When I was speaking to a group of dietitians two years earlier, I heard over and over that people are confused about their food—and a big part of that is not knowing how it is produced. "Where does our food come from? How can we trust it if we don't know who is producing it and what they are doing?" asked a registered dietitian in the first year of her career.

I thought, "Isn't it common sense that ranchers and farm families are growing the plants and animals to feed you?"

I have come to understand the people—and stories—of agriculture are common sense to me because I grew up in agriculture. My roots are firmly planted in the world where food is grown.

Two-thirds of the U.S. population is in cities. Many have never even visited a ranch or a farm. The majority of the Canadian and U.S. population is three to four generations removed from the farm. They have no idea how the food they eat each day is produced until someone tells them. Hence the confusion—and the opportunity to easily buy into misinformation.

The moms at the table told me, "You really need to write a book about this. We want to know what you buy at the grocery, so make it a book we can take to the store with us so we can use it when we're buying food."

I realized there aren't books out there from a rancher's or farmer's perspective actually taking you behind the scenes of today's agriculture in the United States and Canada. We need a book that lifts the curtain on the people growing food, how they do it, and why they are in farming and ranching.

WHY THIS BOOK?

I have an abundantly "full life" between being a mom, running a business that requires a lot of travel, caring for a loved one with cancer, tending to cattle, volunteering, and so on. Adding another project to my to-do list was not a priority. Yet I couldn't stop thinking about what those women said, knowing they represented millions who want, need, and deserve to feel good about the food they buy. In order for that to happen, they need to know the truths from the people who are growing their food, to understand and trust it.

It became too important of an issue for me to ignore. I've had a firsthand perspective of the families growing your food for 40 years.

So I wrote this book—not because I want to push my farm views on you. Not because I need my name on a cover. Not because I believe I have all of the answers.

I do offer a viewpoint that is contrarian to fashionable food; one to help you trust the intentions and process in farming and ranching. I wrote this book because I care about honoring the truth. I care about choice—both on the plate *and* on the farm. I care about parents not feeling guilty when they go to the grocery store and can't afford the "right" label. I care about people not being judged because of what is on their plate or in their grocery bag. I care how instant experts are disparaging farmers and ranchers without knowing what they're talking about. I care that time-crunched parents can buy food—regardless of the brand—with confidence it is safe. I care about children understanding marketing of their food and knowing the real truth in how food is raised. I care about getting back to the truth in food—raised the right way by the right people for the right reasons.

If taking the time to read this book helps you buy, prepare, and enjoy food with confidence—my work translating farm to food will be worth it. I hope you'll keep it in your kitchen as a reference.

After a lifetime as a farm girl and 15 years of working as a professional speaker to bring people together around the plate, I thought the confusion and emotional hysteria around food would die down. I hoped the activists manipulating food companies and consumer minds would move on. I expected journalists with no agricultural background would be called out for their one-sided writing. I assumed people would see through marketing claims being made on food labels. I figured facts would prevail over shoddy science.

I was wrong.

The confusion and emotional battleground continue. The marketing is getting bigger. The misinformation grows. Activists continue to bully. Celebrities and politicians take opinion-based positions instead of looking at the facts. As a result of all of this, food buyers are filled with guilt, confusion, and feelings of being overwhelmed. And the people growing food are left to wonder what happened.

The food hysteria is not going away; it's getting worse.

HOW IS THIS BOOK ORGANIZED?

Food Truths from Farm to Table walks you through aisles of the grocery store, from eggs to cereals to the deli. I outlined these sections for practical purposes of creating a visual of your food shopping experience, then wrote chapters around the most significant issues found in my research. 25 food truths are embedded throughout the book. These food truths are a result of the questions I've fielded from a variety of audiences and know people need answered about their food. The 25 truths are also what I believe are at the heart of the divide between food and farm.

This book brings a voice of reason to the overly sensationalized food and health arena. My hope is that food truths from the people producing your food are a valuable and unique perspective. I want to arm you with the truths about food to simplify your food-buying experience. My goal is to provide practical evidence in an emotional arena often filled with knee-jerk reactions. You may not agree with everything I write—and that's okay; I welcome debate.

This book will give you a different window into the food world to simplify your food shopping, reduce your guilt, and give you freedom to enjoy food. May this book help you turn food confusion into clarity so you have confidence that the food you buy, prepare, and serve to your family is safe, healthy, and nourishing.

25 Food Truths to Shop & Eat without Guilt

1. Hormones are in everything.
2. Antibiotics have benefits.
3. Animal welfare is an hourly concern on farms and ranches.
4. Housing is used to protect animals—and your food—from nature.
5. Organic farming is about production methods, not nutritional value.
6. Marketing on labels is confusing consumers.
7. Food costs are a shared concern.
8. Local is not always better for the environment.
9. Chemicals are naturally in food and are needed to protect it.
10. Genes are the coolest ingredient on your plate.
11. Food safety starts on the farm and ends in your kitchen.
12. Sustainability is complex and essential to family businesses.
13. Food is an amazing science from farm to table.
14. The answer to food waste is hidden in your refrigerator.
15. Soil is a farm's greatest asset.
16. Grains are an important part of your diet.
17. Sugar, salt, and moderation are a natural part of a balanced diet.
18. Fat isn't always bad.
19. Corn is tasty—and healthy—for animals and people.
20. Hypocrisy happens in food, health, and nutrition.
21. Convenience is reality; it's not always wrong or right.
22. Choice on the farm and choice on the plate involve a balancing act.

23. Pay less now, and pay more later in your health.
24. The media isn't the best source of information about food.
25. Buying and eating the right food doesn't have to be time consuming.

1

Take Guilt Off Your Food List

WHAT'S YOUR CHEETOS?

A couple of years ago, my daughter and two of our closest friends went on a week-long spring break vacation to Tempe, Arizona. My 11-year-old daughter and I were both up before sunrise because our bodies were still on Eastern Time.

We moved stealthily through the dark hotel room we were sharing with friends in search of our vacation tradition. My daughter found the bag on the shelf by the TV and giggled. We both jumped back in bed. I tried to open the bag as quietly as possible. Then we discovered Cheetos are never quiet when you have room-mates! As we munched (somewhat loudly) on our vacation breakfast of Cheetos, our friends woke up in disbelief.

"What is that noise?" Jenny and Ellie asked. They looked over and caught us crunching on Cheetos and licking our orange fingertips. "Two health freaks are eating CHEETOS? For breakfast? In bed? Wait 'til we tell everyone about this!"

Let's just say our decade-long friends were shocked to see us lounge in bed glee-fully eating junk food for breakfast. Apparently they were not aware: I happily pack some variation of cheese puffs for every vacation. My daughter reminds me. Every trip. And then we laugh while munching away and trying to get the Cheetos crumbs out of the bed.

I am an advocate for healthy eating. The majority of the time I am committed to providing healthy meals for my family. Our pantry doesn't have a lot of junk food; I work hard to cook tasty and nutritious food. My daughter has a protein, vegetable, and fruit for lunch and dinner. She has milk at every meal and willingly chooses it over soda at restaurants. I work out three times per week and she ran in the state cross-country meet as a sixth grader. We are not perfect, but we do try to be healthy like most average active families.

But I also believe food is a celebration, designed to bring people together. Food is a big part of our family traditions.

The orange fingertips and bed crumbs of Cheetos is a fun tradition that my daughter and I relish when we are on vacation. It's a bonding experience. I hope she will always remember our Cheetos moments and pass on our orange-fingertip tradition to her own kids someday.

This may surprise you. It's just that I believe that indulging occasionally in food that is not good for you is good for you—as long as it's done occasionally. Everything in moderation. Our indulgence is balanced with a lot of nutrition the other days of the year, regular exercise, and healthy home-cooked meals.

What's your version of Cheetos? Are you a dad who always buys your growing son a pizza after he plays a basketball game? Do you indulge in beer and brats with your friends every Fourth of July? Do you celebrate Thanksgiving with grandmother's pie, gravy, and all the fixings? Are your holidays filled with cookies? Food is central to these celebrations; food is designed to bring people together.

After all, food is meant to be enjoyed. Food provides nourishment. Food is a basic necessity.

Give up the guilt about an occasional "bad" food. To paraphrase the Shakespeare quote, "Food is not good or bad, but thinking makes it so."

We live in an era of food judgment . . . feed your baby organic baby food if you want to be a "good" mother, buy local if you're a "true" foodie, make sure you have the right brand on your bag, and only invite friends to the trendiest restaurants where you can philosophize over food origins. Large is bad, small is good—in food portions, farm size, business, and waistlines. Technology in food production is frowned upon. And anyone with a vested interest in agriculture is surely so biased, they can't be trusted.

Frankly, it's tiring. Food is food. You eat and so do I. What one family consumes does not make them superior or inferior. The same is true in farming; the way one family farms does not make them worthy of accolades or condemnation. It's about choice. And like many things in life, not everyone makes the same choices.

JUDGING THE SOUL OF FOOD

It seems we have moved beyond mere concern about our food to judging the soul of food—and those who consume it. What is the soul of food? For me, the soul of food has everything to do with beautiful black and white Holsteins gracing my front yard and neighborhood. The soul of food is about the people who painstakingly care for the land and animals so that you can eat. The soul of food is about the memories made around my dining room table with my family and friends.

The soul of food is likely different to you.

Food perspective varies based upon your position around the proverbial plate. Farmers come off as defensive when they refuse to acknowledge that questions have merit and there are other experts in the discussion. They see food as what they do every day and don't understand why there are so many questions. Scientists look to facts; chefs look at the soul of food as how it will add flavor to their creation; dietitians consider health implications; and parents look the convenience, cost, and "feel-good" factor. One perspective is not more superior than the other.

When I wrote my first book, *No More Food Fights!*, it became apparent we would never all agree on the right kind of food or farming style. However, it is time for us to stop the judgment on food. Food judgment and food elitists should not trump realism in the soul of food.

In other words, don't let "judgment on food soul" overcome "soul of food." Your choices differ from mine. A single mom trying to make ends meet has different wants than a Whole Foods follower. A dietitian concerned with a balanced diet has different food priorities than a middle-aged man looking for comfort food.

I don't believe any of those people have a more superior food soul. A Super Bowl ad does not make the soul of food, a celebrity sensationalizing food claims does not make the soul of food, the words on a label do not make the soul of food, nor does a fad diet. All are what I call food soul judgments. All lead to food elitism and, consequently, food shaming.

In reality, the soul of food today is largely the same as it was 50 years ago. Food is, in fact, safer—but I recognize facts don't create the perceived soul of food. If you have a romanticized view of small family farms with crops raised by hand and animals lovingly running free while eating green grass, you may be surprised by the reality of farming with animals in mud, sweating it out while pulling weeds from crops, and trying to eek a living out of the land.

We've allowed individual judgment of food to dictate the soul of food over the last decade. Food is not a religion, nor should a tribe be dictating what is right for your family. The soul of my food is no different from the soul of your food.

What matters is how food nourishes a family.

Join me in a trip around the grocery store to be armed with 25 truths you urgently need to know about food so you can shop without guilt, confusion, or judgment. Learn the truths so you can recognize marketing and move on.

Part I: Dairy

Milk was once considered the standby beverage of choice to grow healthy kids. Now questions abound about whether milk is making our kids fat, causing breast development by first grade, or adding antibiotics to our diet. The truths inside the dairy case may surprise you!

"If you change the way you look at things, the things you look at change."
—Wayne Dyer

2. Are Happy Cows on Drugs Harming My Kids?

CALVES, KIDS, AND COW TIPPING

Calves happily munched on sweet grain while the sun filtered in the wooden barn doors as dust rose up from the broom I was running down the center aisle while chattering with the "babies." Those sweet little black and white calves with wet noses and tongues longer than my arms created my earliest childhood memories.

Since those days of doing chores in my parents' red and white calf barn, I've visited hundreds of dairy farms, large and small, in a dozen countries. It takes a special soul to be a dairy farmer. It is a profession that is "on call" 24/7 by animals who don't say thank you for tender loving care and interrupt the best-laid plans to go to a family gathering.

What do you see when you stand at the dairy case? I see black and white cows known as Holsteins. I see my first calf, "Bambi"—several hundred pounds of pure stubbornness delivering lessons in tenacity when I was nine years old and scared of her. I see Perfect, whom I purchased for $7,000 when I was 12 years old. We took home several trophies together, and her offspring later paid for my college education.

And when I am at the dairy case, I see Lucky, my daughter's sweet black calf who gleefully reached her head and long tongue through the gate at the state fair to greet people. I think about standing in our pasture and watching that beautiful black calf and blonde girl learn life lessons together.

My situation is not unusual—dairy farmers across the country have stories like this, too. But I also know these images are unique to people from a dairy farm, so I understand you may not see those cattle in the dairy case. The choice of 1 percent, 2 percent, whole milk, vitamin D, hormones or not, and about 25 other label claims make it confusing. Overwhelming. More than what any food buyer needs.

While I realize you'll likely never think of Bambi, Perfect, and Lucky, I would like to clear up the dairy case confusion. Just to address a few dairy case myths: cows are not happier in one state versus another (e.g., California Happy Cows), dairy cattle are not starving because you can see their bones (think figure skaters, not hockey players), you cannot tip a cow (you will likely end up kicked), and farmers are not pumping cows full of drugs.

The big questions and food myths:
- *Does milk have hormones in it?*
- *Should I be worried about hormones in milk?*
- *Why even drink milk?*

HORMONE-FREE FOOD?

Do you enjoy the thought of hormones? As a woman, I don't care for hormones dancing through my body. As a mom, I worry about my little girl developing early because of hormones. As a breeder of those pretty black and white dairy cows you see on food labels, I have great respect for hormones.

My respect for hormones comes from watching a favorite cow giving birth to a beautiful newborn 90-pound calf. It's amazing to witness the reproductive cycle, from the breeding of a cow to the birthing of a calf. It takes education and experience to understand the special care a 1,500-pound cow requires during her pregnancy. Hormones allow all of that to happen—they make it possible to breed more cattle. The end result? More milk and meat for you.

That's why hormones in food don't freak me out. It's different when you see hormones in action on a daily basis while working with plants and animals. If you or your friends have had fertility assistance in having a family, such as in vitro fertilization, you benefited from the extensive reproductive work done in bovines, as cattle reproductive systems are remarkably similar to humans. Yet there is this fear of hormones from milk.

While I was at a party at one of my friend's homes, another mom proudly exclaimed, "I'm really careful to give my kids hormone-free food."

I tried not to cringe, asking her as kindly as I could, "Do you really believe your food is healthier?"

"Well, the label says 'hormone free.'" Then I asked her if the breast milk she had fed her kids when they were babies was hormone free.

"No way, not with all the hormones raging through my body," was her immediate answer. The light went on . . . and all I had to say was, "Cows have those same hormones. They always have. All of your food has hormones in it, regardless of label claims."

Food labels claiming "hormone free" are lies. All milk has hormones in it; it always has. It always will or it would not exist. Do not let marketing hysteria sway you otherwise.

HORMONE HYSTERIA STARTED ON A LABEL

Hormones are a natural part of our world—they are required for living. *Merriam-Webster* defines hormone as a product of living cells that circulates in body fluids (as blood) or sap and produces a specific, often stimulatory, effect on the activity of cells, usually remote from its point of origin.

In other words, hormones are required for life. Yet hormones have become akin to a nasty four-letter word in food. Why? They exist in every plant and animal you eat. Minerals like salt are the exception. You are consuming hormones at every meal unless you have a salt lollipop. Using the definition, maple syrup could be called hormone juice since it's the sap of a tree filled with hormones.

It's a fascinating marketing case study to look at how fear is used to scare people into changing their food purchases. The hysteria around "hormones in dairy products" is a prime example. Labels are often used to convey a claim to alter the perception of the product in order for the manufacturer and retailer to sell more or sell at a higher price.

For example, consider the fear mongering around the protein hormone recombinant bovine somatotropin (rbST), which was approved by the Food and Drug Administration (FDA) in 1993 and entered the marketplace. I have personal familiarity with rbST from my days working as an undergraduate in the Animal Reproductive Physiology Laboratory at Michigan State University. I gave a lot of cows shots of rbST. I can tell you without question when the cows are properly cared for (dairy people call this management), rbST doesn't hurt them.

Why? Because bST naturally occurs in their body—it's necessary for the production of milk—just like somatotropins are present in all animals (including women) with lactating capabilities. Somatotropin is a protein hormone that is important to support tissue health, growth, and maintenance. Giving a cow a "booster" means she will make about 7 percent more milk—and will require more food (think of an Olympic athlete burning more calories) to sustain the right body weight. The resulting milk is the same; there is no test that has identified additional hormone levels from cows given rbST—and only about 15 percent of dairy farmers choose to use rbST.

You may also hear about insulin-like growth factor I (IGF-I), a protein hormone controlled by bST, being higher in cows given rbST. Here's what you need to know: IGF-I levels in milk from rbST-supplemented cows are within the normal range and are lower than levels found naturally in human blood and other tissues. It's important to understand this protein hormone is safe, even in high doses.[1] Like any other dietary proteins, enzymes in your digestive tract break down all protein hormones—such as bST and IGF-I—before you absorb them.

HORMONES AND BROKEN BONES—THROUGH THE EYES OF A HEALTH PROFESSIONAL

Do hormones have benefits? Sure! A dietary protein, like milk, benefits bones partially because of its ability to increase IGF-I, which supports bone formation.[2]

It's a health risk to avoid milk because hormones or other claims around "humans drinking cows' milk" have made the headlines. As a registered nurse from Ohio, Mary Fleming, said, "We use the technology of recombinant DNA to make Humulin insulin for our human patients. And we celebrate that! We are just using the same technology when we use rbST—and it means that there is a much lower environmental impact of feeding people. I'm a nurse with a master's degree in public health who has studied the issue. Please drink the milk to prevent osteoporosis, which is a MUCH bigger problem than hormones. Seventy-five percent of women and 50 percent of men do not get adequate calcium in their diet. Dairy products cannot be matched for the available calcium by other foods or supplements. Furthermore, a huge percentage of the people who fracture their hips due to osteoporosis will die within a year."

People are missing out on the benefits of milk because of hormone claims. Keep in mind the FDA found there was no significant difference between milk from supplemented and unsupplemented cows, so it did not have the authority to require such labeling. That label claims are not related to a meaningful difference in the milk's composition is supported by research published in the *Journal of the American Dietetic Association*. This is the reason that if any milk processor makes a claim on the package about not using artificial hormones, the claim must have an asterisk with the following statement: "The FDA has determined that no significant difference has been shown between milk derived from rbST-supplemented and non-rbST-supplemented cows."

DO DAIRY PRODUCTS MAKE GIRLS DEVELOP EARLIER?

I've never met a parent who doesn't worry about their children—especially when it comes to hormones.

"There are naturally occurring hormones in all foods, including breast milk. Plants like soybeans and cabbage contain hormones. Meat and milk have small quantities of hormones, but at levels far lower than what humans produce in their own bodies on a daily basis," according to Dr. Ann Pacrina of Penn State University. If you still question the role of hormones, check the hormone levels in women's breast milk.

There is no scientific proof about consumption of milk causing early puberty, whether from cows supplemented with rbST or naturally containing bST, or other hormones.[3] The Academy of Nutrition and Dietetics (AND) reported that girls enter puberty today at a younger age than they did 30 years ago. There is debate as to how much earlier, but studies indicate it is only six months earlier.

Some scientists believe the increase in childhood obesity may lead to earlier puberty. Dr. Biro from the University of Cincinnati points out a fattier diet and more food may be largely responsible for girls developing earlier. Observational studies link higher body mass index or increased body fatness with earlier puberty.[4]

Consider this: puberty is the preparation of the body to begin supporting reproduction. A body that has received more nutrition over the course of time reaches that point earlier. Fattier foods mean a body reaches that point earlier.

Again, as a mom, I don't relish the thought of hormones in my daughter's body—nor am I particularly fond of the hormonal highs and lows of adolescence.

But it's comforting to know milk, cheese, Greek yogurt, and other dairy products in our refrigerator do not amplify my child's hormones.

HORMONES ARE NOT A HEALTH CONCERN

I understand the concerns you have about feeding your family. If you're convinced buying milk produced in a certain way is best for your family—it is absolutely okay. Please just know labels are marketing tools, and EVERY product in the dairy case has similar levels of hormones in it, including extracts from almond and soybeans, marketed as "almond milk" or "soy milk." Plant-based products like almond and soy milk are actually higher in estrogen and progesterone than cow's milk.

I'm not knocking nuts or soybeans; just be clear that hormones happen in BOTH plants and animals. Per the definition—a "hormone produces a specific, often stimulatory, effect on the activity of cells." bST occurs in cows naturally to help them produce milk. The same with reproductive hormones like estrogen, testosterone, and progesterone; hormones are a part of that miraculous cycle I described at the beginning of the chapter. Just like your body has those same hormones at work—it's called life.

Farmers—and consumers—have their freedom of choice removed when marketing trumps science. Such was the case with milk label claims targeting foodie consumers of the Northeast, which started with concerns about hormones in milk. Retailer-differentiation thought labeling milk "hormone free" would attract more customers. More customers mean more money. As such, it became fashionable to put hormone claims on milk.

Hormones happen. Hormones are NOT the bad guys—and they've always been a part of your food. Don't be lulled into marketing mania or mistruths. Hormones are not the boogeyman lurking in the dairy case, waiting to reach out and grab you by the neck as soon as you reach for a gallon of milk without the right label!

It's not just my opinion; scientific evidence does not show the presence of hormones in cow's milk is a health concern.[5] The World Health Organization (WHO), National Institutes of Health (NIH), FDA and other country's scientific bodies have all said rbST is safe. You may not be a big believer in federal standards, but a healthy dose of respect should be given to the rigorous process and incredible scrutiny of products being used in food production. Hormones, as well as antibiotics and other products used to keep cows healthy and productive, are part of the FDA's food safety evaluation.

The labels known as "absence claims" should be titled "guilt laden labels," in my opinion—for example, milk labeled with hormone, natural, or antibiotic claims. There are as many claims about milk as there are products in the dairy case.

GOT NUTRITION?

However, nutrition counts. Milk is critical for long-term health. Dairy products are one of the most powerful nutritional tools. Starting at age nine, girls are getting fewer dairy products than recommended during their lifetime.[6] The same is true for the male side of the population, beginning around age 19. At that point, men begin being at least a cup short of dairy compared to the guidelines.

The bottom line is this: you need the calcium, and there is no better source than milk that allows your body to absorb calcium. All milk has hormones—and there is no test to detect any supplemented hormones since they naturally occur in a milking female.

Milk hasn't changed a whole lot over the years, aside from reducing fat, increasing protein, and improving food safety. Food science research has resulted in adding a whole lot more cool products, like Greek yogurt, to the dairy case. Dairy products pack minerals and vitamins that are essential to your health—don't let half-truths about hormones dissuade you from doing dairy.

The International Food Information Council (IFIC) brings insight to your dairy case dilemma. "A recent study published in the Journal of the Academy of Nutrition and Dietetics (AND) looked at the quality, nutritional value and hormone composition of milk purchased at retail stores that were labeled according to farm-management practice—organic, processor-certified as not from cows supplemented with rbST, or conventional.

The study found that the type of label was not related to any meaningful differences in nutritional value, quality, or hormone composition. The hormones measured were bovine somatotropin, IGF-1, progesterone and estradiol. The authors conclude that "it is important for food and nutrition professionals to know that conventional, rbST-free and organic milk are compositionally similar so they can serve as a key resource to consumers who are making milk purchase (and consumption) decisions in a marketplace where there are misleading milk label claims."[7]

Disregard the label claims and enjoy your dairy products.

3. Your Milk Is Not Filled with Antibiotics

THE SCIENCE OF ANIMAL CARE

Peppermint has always had a special place in our heart. One of the cutest calves I've seen, she was born at Christmas time with a whole lot of fuzzy hair and immediately looking for attention from us. She's sassy, sweet, and pretty. Peppermint has a special relationship with my daughter and

Food Truth
Antibiotics have benefits.

seems to have an innate knowledge to be very careful with kids who come visit. One summer day in July, she lay in the pasture with five kiddos on her back while she chewed her cud, seemingly smiling. Needless to say, she is spoiled—especially as one of the last few descendants of my Perfect cow family.

Like every other dairy cow, Peppermint was bred so she could begin producing milk around two years of age. That is the purpose of dairy cattle. We were hoping she'd have a heifer (female calf), but those hopes came to an end as she showed signs of calving (giving birth) a few weeks early. My dairy farmer neighbor and I agreed there was little chance of the calf being alive. We do everything we can to save calves, but there is no special neonatal intensive care unit (NICU) for premature calves; they rarely make it.

As my daughter stood by Peppermint's head on a cold February night, I pulled out a backwards female calf (they're usually born front legs first, with their head tucked between the legs). The heifer was dead, and Peppermint delivered the dead twin bull (male) later that night on her own. Even though we knew not to expect a live birth, it was still a letdown. My daughter, then 10, said, "It's OK, as long as Peppermint is good."

Unfortunately, dead animals are a part of farming. So is dealing with sick cattle, which can be incredibly frustrating—especially when a little girl's only wish is for her animal to be healthy. Cows who deliver dead calves often have problems with a uterine infection and require treatment with antibiotics. A farmer has to have a Rolodex of mental medical knowledge and a good veterinarian to effectively treat animals. It would be cruel to withhold those from an animal in pain, and the milk is not put into the bulk tank. We call keeping the milk out "withholding"— it is required when antibiotics are used to treat sick dairy cattle—and it means that the milk does not enter the food supply.

We also gave her vitamins, probiotics, painkillers, and microbials. Unfortunately, she just stopped eating and no one could find an answer. In two weeks' time, Peppermint went from being a strong healthy animal to nearly dying and stumping the veterinarians at Purdue University's Large Animal Clinic.

As I stood at Peppermint's side giving her an IV before I drove her in a trailer hitched to a truck up to Purdue, I couldn't help but wonder how many animal rights activists have cried as they tried to find answers to make sick animals better. It made me angry to think how inauthentic it is for well-funded activist groups such as People for the Ethical Treatment of Animals (PETA) and the Human Society of the United States (HSUS) to make claims when they have never had blood- and manure-stained hands from helping sick farm animals.

The big questions and food myths:

- *Are there antibiotics in dairy products?*
- *Why do farmers give cows antibiotics?*
- *Is it really safe and important to drink milk?*

CARING FOR ANIMALS WITH A CONSCIENCE

Science ended up on Peppermint's side. She had two transfusions of rumen "bugs" at the veterinary clinic. These bugs are actually bacteria—the good kind—that jump-started her rumen, which is the most important part of a cow's stomach. Cows have complex digestive systems, and rumen health is key to cow health. The bacteria for the transfusion were collected from a fistulated cow, which is a research cow with a surgically placed permanent access portal (a sealed hole) to her rumen. The fistulated cow lives pain free; her tissue grows around the portal, and collecting rumen bugs is as easy as opening a window and reaching in.

The transfusion of rumen bacteria from that cow to Peppermint saved her life. She started eating again and came back to the dairy farm, though her milk continued to be withheld for the FDA-mandated time for the antibiotic she was given. Then her milk was tested before it was put in the tank on the farm to ensure there were no residuals in it. Next, milk from the bulk tank was tested before it was put on the truck. Finally, milk was tested again at the processing plant. You get the idea!

Peppermint went back to her ornery self, much to our relief. She has since had two healthy heifer calves, was reserve Grand Champion at our county fair, and received a lot of love in the meantime. Her purpose is still to produce milk, and she will eventually be food, but I'm so thankful she recovered and my daughter's wish was granted.

You see, people who care for animals do so with a conscience—we consider it an honor and privilege to do so. We give medication accordingly—with a conscience. Yes, Peppermint is a cow with a name in an average-size herd of cows. However, farm size doesn't change the care, concern, and human conscience that go into responsible animal care. If you've ever stood with a farm animal and cried because you felt so incredibly frustrated about not being able to make the animal feel better, you'd know why we want and need every tool available—including antibiotics.

Antibiotics are most commonly used in dairy cattle to treat mastitis infections. Mastitis is an inflammation and infection of the mammary gland—and it can be incredibly painful, as any mom who has experienced it can explain. Depending on the type of mastitis, the udder may swell up, the cow can have a fever, or in the worst cases, the infection becomes systemic, endangering the cow's life. This is not due to unsanitary conditions, stressed cattle, overmilking, or "factory farms"—just like it is not a human's fault when she gets mastitis. Some animals are just more prone to getting this infection, and the best prevention in the world can't keep every cow from getting mastitis—even though farmers try their best.

Antibiotics are reserved for use when an animal needs to be treated; the approved treatments for this infection are expensive and this means that milk from that cow cannot be sold, which adds up to a double expense to the farm. Given the extremely low profit margins in dairy farming and the farmer's commitment to doing the right thing for their animals, a lot of precautions are taken to eliminate all controllable mastitis cases. However, antibiotics do have benefits—they help a sick animal (human, cow, or monkey) fight off infection.

Cows injected with antibiotics may carry some residue of the antibiotic in their milk, just like you secrete medication through your tears, saliva, and urine. Milk from treated cows is withheld—it is not put into the bulk tank with the rest of the herd's milk. It is discarded. Care is taken to ensure milk from treated cows does not have any impact on the other milk, such as rinsing milkers (milking machines) and lines that the withheld milk traveled down to be removed from the system.

Why do we even milk cows with mastitis? Milking gets the bad cells out of the cow's udder to reduce the infection. It's also important for a cow's comfort.

Milk is not allowed to contain any detectable antibiotics. The FDA Grade A Pasteurized Milk Ordinance, revised in 2009, has a legal standard requiring milk to contain no detectable antibiotics when analyzed using approved test methods. Interestingly, the Pasteurized Milk Ordinance dates back to 1924. If you're buying milk in the grocery store, the only kind you're purchasing is Grade A.

As a side note, let's look at how much safer milk has become as a result of the ordinance. In 1938, milk-borne outbreaks constituted 25 percent of all disease outbreaks due to infected foods and contaminated water. Now milk and fluid milk products continue to be associated with less than 1 percent of such reported outbreaks.[8]

When antibiotics are used responsibly, they do not enter your food supply. Milk is tested multiple times to be sure no milk enters the food supply with antibiotics in it. Milk goes from the cow through a milking machine to a bulk tank, where it is chilled. Milk samples are taken from the farm's bulk tank for antibiotic residue testing before being loaded on to a tanker. Every tanker of milk in the United States is also tested before the milk is pumped from the tanker for delivery at the processing plant. If the milk passes the test, it is pumped into the plant's holding tanks for processing, such as pasteurization, homogenization, or being turned into cheese, ice cream, yogurt, etc.

If milk does not pass antibiotic testing, the entire tanker load of milk is discarded. Farm samples are then reviewed to find the source of the antibiotic residues. The farm is usually held financially responsible for the entire tanker full of milk, fines can be involved, and the processor may refuse shipment in the future. The veterinarian for the farm is also contacted and may be put under review by the FDA. As any dairy farmer or veterinarian will tell you, antibiotics are NOT something they take lightly.

This gets back to the common sense thing. It seems like common sense to a farmer caring for animals that we will not pump expensive antibiotics in them to poison the milk supply, pay penalties, and potentially lose the right to ship milk. However, since most people haven't milked cows, I have come to understand this may not be common sense in the grocery store.

WHY DOES MILK MATTER?

Last week we were out of milk so I stopped by the local gas station to get some on my way home from a business trip. "People still drink this stuff?" asked the attendant as I paid.

I was a bit flabbergasted, but managed to get out, "Yes, it's kind of essential for calcium and a bunch of other nutrients." Judging from his response, he wasn't terribly concerned about nutrition, but the episode did leave me scratching my head. Cheese, yogurt, ice cream, sour cream, and milk are staples in my fridge, and milk is served at every meal in my house.

The American Academy of Pediatrics states, "Strong evidence exists regarding the benefit from consuming a diet rich in low or nonfat milk and other dairy products."[9] The AND also says, "The fortification of milk with vitamin D has virtually eliminated the risk of vitamin D deficiency in children. However, the rising consumption of juice and soft drinks in place of milk is increasing the probability of deficiency, which can lead to rickets or defective bone growth."[10]

Calcium, other minerals, and vitamins are best absorbed from real food, like dairy products. You're not going to find a better way to take care of your bones than dairy. Besides the calcium, milk also provides protein, riboflavin, vitamins A and D, phosphorus, potassium, magnesium, and other vitamins and minerals.

The *Dietary Guidelines* are issued and updated every five years by the U.S. Department of Agriculture (USDA) and the U.S. Department of Health and Human Services. These guidelines show dairy is:

- Responsible for improved bone health and may reduce the risk of osteoporosis.
- Important to bone health during childhood and adolescence, when bone mass is being built.
- Associated with a reduced risk of cardiovascular disease and type 2 diabetes and with lower blood pressure in adults.

In other words, your body needs dairy. It's critical for growth, which is why milk, cheese, yogurt, cottage cheese, and other dairy products are REALLY important for kids. It saddens me to read about toddlers becoming ill after drinking soda, almond milk, and soy milk—a disturbing trend today. Kids of all ages need dairy!

4. Animal Welfare Is 24-Hour Care

BOVINE BREAST PUMPS

"Why does she look so happy?" my friend Lisa asked as she watched the cow visibly relax and her eyes droop happily. "Did you ever use a breast pump?" I asked. Lisa was slightly appalled, but came back with, "Yes. Why?"

"Remember how it felt when you really needed that pump? That's how she feels—relief and satisfaction." We were standing in the barn at the fairgrounds on a hot July night. As 4-H members buzzed around, we were watching my daughter milk Peppermint after a show—which you can think of as a cow beauty pageant. The cow's reaction was almost as though she had just had a massage at the world's best spa—a look of pure contentment.

> **Food Truth**
>
> Animal welfare is an hourly concern on farms and ranches.

In some ways, cows are not so different from other animals. They have big personalities, are creatures of habit, and have huge expressive eyes—kind of like your dog. But they're not dogs—dairy cattle weigh up to a ton, drink a bathtub of water a day, and are designed to provide us with food.

After a lifetime with dairy cattle, I can tell you it is an honor and privilege to care for them. Cows are milked to provide nutritious food, not because we are cruel, but because that is their purpose.

The big questions and food myths:

- *Do farmers abuse their animals?*
- *Isn't it cruel to put cows in barns?*
- *Why are calves taken away from their moms?*

MOMS, KIDS, AND CONFINED COWS

A fellow professional speaker taught me the value of firsthand perspective on concerns about farming practices. She visited a modern farm, where she went from being a skeptic of modern agriculture to finding moms just like her. Eliz Greene, a spokesperson for the American Heart Association, shared the eye-opening experience she had when she visited a dairy farm:

> Ever wonder where your milk comes from? I got a chance to find out when I visited a dairy farm in western Wisconsin.
> Having only the media view of "factory" farming, I was firmly on the organic/ free range/family farm side of the argument and a little concerned about visiting a

large farm. I have to say my view has changed—I still need more info, but it isn't as black and white as I thought. I visited a dairy farm with more than 800 cows—which is huge. It is run by a family (two brothers and their wives) and some employees (total of 12 people I think). They'd like to have more help, but can't afford them with the low milk prices.

I had assumed "confined" cows would be unhappy cows, dirty cows, sad cows—but I was wrong. Over the hour-long tour, our host constantly talked about "cow comfort" from the different types of bedding to how the feed was presented. They invest in various types of fans and misters to keep the cows cool—they even had motion-sensitive back scratching machines for the cows. It was a bit uncomfortable to watch one cow use it—she seemed to be REALLY enjoying it.

As anyone who has breastfed knows, if the mom is stressed or uncomfortable, the milk doesn't flow. I hadn't considered this concept in regard to dairy cows, but it makes sense. From that perspective, it seems ridiculous that a business person would set up a situation where conditions would limit production. No, indeed—this farm was all about making the cows happy.

Our host talked about his routine, and it was obvious how hard they work and they are struggling to make a profit. With their cute little kids running around it is hard to believe this was what an article in *Time Magazine* had called a "soulless" operation. Instead, I found moms I could relate to.

Here's what I've learned from my time on the farm:

- The farmers I met are VERY busy, care deeply, and deserve our respect.
- There's more to this issue than I ever imagined.
- I don't know enough yet—it is time to get more information and start really understanding where our food comes from.

I suspect there is more than one right answer, and the people who are most qualified to help me understand are the people working hard to produce our food.

It's amazing how visiting a farm can build understanding, isn't it? Eliz found moms like her, except their children were in the barn. She could relate to the women through a shared perspective. Farmers are humans, too. Families are the fabric of our world—and at the heart of farming and ranching.

IT'S PERSONAL TO A DAIRY FARMER

We, as farmers, take our work so personally that it leads us to become defensive at times, particularly when we are feeling attacked. Farming is a way of life, as well as our family business—it's difficult for us to differentiate the people and practices. As such, when farming practices are being questioned, the farmer feels he is being questioned himself.

One of the questions that often comes up is why cows are so skinny. It's a simple answer. Dairy cattle are skinny not because they are being abused, but it's in their genes to turn calories into milk. They're like Olympic athletes. Dairy cattle on grass would be akin to Michael Phelps only eating lettuce and veggies instead of the 12,000 calories he consumed each day when he was in training. Dairy cattle typically have half grain and half forage (grassy or hay) diets to meet their caloric needs.

Cows have four compartments to their stomach, with a large fermentation area known as the rumen. There are bacteria in the rumen (think about Peppermint's story of rumen bugs), allowing cows to get nutrition from cellulose and fibrous material that humans can't. It's also why cows are recyclers of many by-product feeds, such as corn gluten, soybean meal, almond hulls, etc. How do you know a ruminant? Look for them chewing their cud—it's actually regurgitated feed. Gross, but useful in digestion.

As mentioned, it is an honor and a privilege to care for dairy cattle. Dairy farming involves millions of dollars of risk (due to the capital required for facilities, feed, etc.), grueling work at all hours of the day and night, and taking what price is given to you by the processor in a fluctuating market. People don't milk cows because they want to abuse them or take advantage of them for pure profit; farmers do so because they love dairy cattle.

Are there dairy farmers who don't take good care of their animals? Sure—just like there are teachers who abuse children, clergy who make terrible choices, and executives who embezzle millions. Thankfully, abusive farmers are in the distinct minority because they can't stay in business long; you cannot abuse an animal and expect it to make milk for you.

UNDERSTANDING THE CONTEXT OF ANIMAL CARE

What's one of the greatest challenges for the good guys—those who are trying to take care of their cattle? Many images are taken out of context by animal rights activists and splashed throughout the media. If you've never been on a dairy farm, you may not understand why we take a calf away from the mother cow or dehorn a calf.

Dehorning is an example of a necessary animal care practice that can look ugly. Horns are removed from a calf's head, which looks and sounds cruel. Yet, dehorning is a critical safety practice. Cattle with horns can gore each other. Just as importantly, they can gore our family members. Farmers prefer gentle dispositions in animals and work with animals to create an environment comfortable for them, but safety is a priority.

A mean cow is not anything you want to mess with; they will toss a human body into the air, stick their horns in when the body slams to the ground, and then smash it with their head. If that image isn't attractive, remember dehorning protects humans and animals. It's not a matter of farm size or how an animal is housed; accidents with cattle injuring humans happen in pasture and pens.

Have you ever breastfed or been head butted by a baby head? If so, you may have more of an understanding about how much damage a 100-pound calf can do to a cow's udder. Calves slam the udder, which is not only painful to the cow, but also can cause mastitis. Additionally, calves can damage the teats, making the cow more susceptible to disease. Separation is best for both—it also allows the calf's diet to be closely monitored.

This is a different story than what animal rights organizations claim about practices to keep animals—and our families—safe. Like most animal lovers, I find it hard to resist a fuzzy little kitten or puppy dog playing. My childhood memories revolve around animals—trying to persuade the Saint Bernard to pull me on a sled, raising orphan kittens, and having calves as playmates. I also recall going to local animal shelters as a child and feeling terrible for the animals that had no home, so I understand the attraction to campaigns run by the HSUS.

The reality is that HSUS advertises to attract animal lovers' dollars. Many great people and organizations have contributed because they want to help animals. An *Animal People News* article has shown that HSUS contributes more to its own $11 million pension plan than to local shelters.[11]

Why? Take a look at "The Myth of the Humane Society of the United States," a law school article that outlines how the bulk of the HSUS's income was spent on fundraising, campaigns, and lawsuits: "There is one minor detail left out of these commercials. HSUS is not a large network of animal shelters, as it would have you believe. In fact, the HSUS does not own, operate, or lease a single animal shelter in our country."[12]

Contrast this type of political activity to that of people who work with animals every day. It's similar to the debate around government and education. Do you trust the people who are working with students daily to deliver education the most effectively—or those who are creating a system? As a mom, I trust teachers trained in education and I expect them to make the best decisions related to education. While I understand the importance of national and state standards, I also see such standards limiting the true experts—teachers—and I value the firsthand expertise of those teachers far more than I trust outside influencers in setting educational standards.

When it comes to farm animals, firsthand expertise means a farmer knows when an animal isn't feeling right by looking in the animal's eye. A farmer determines how to best handle the situation based on experience, data about the animal, and the farmer's ongoing education. Farmers work with experts such as veterinarians and nutritionists, along with state and national organizations, to adhere to best practices as standards, many of which are verified. Just as a reference point, the larger the farm, the greater the regulations and the larger the team of experts helping the farmer.

Farmers are deeply committed to the animals in our care.

Dr. Kathy Swift, a veterinarian, mom, and wife of a grocery store manager, provides insight on proper animal care on a dairy farm, both for animal welfare and business profitability. Swift works with dairies that milk more than 1,000 cows and manage their comfort in extreme heat of Florida.

If you think farmers are driven more by profit than by caring about the well-being of their animals, consider the scientific evidence that clearly shows that a farm's profit suffers if its animals are routinely mistreated because the animals won't grow. And, in Dr. Swift's words, there's more to the story:

Happy cows aren't just an advertising slogan; it's something farmers strive to make happen every day. Growing up on a dairy farm, I still remember that even at a young age, treating animals with kindness and respect was important to the farm's success. It wasn't until years later that I actually learned the science behind the importance of a neighboring farm's mantra, clearly displayed in their barn, "Speak to the cow as if she were a lady." It comes down to the stress hormone, cortisol. Cortisol (known as hydrocortisone when taken as a prescribed anti-inflammatory medication) is activated whenever an animal is under stress. This hormone is very important in that it plays a big part in the "fight or flight" phenomenon. Its release causes a chain reaction that causes the body to raise blood pressure, accelerate the action of the heart and lungs, and dilation of blood vessels going to the muscles.

All of these are important in the animal's ability to protect itself and escape a dangerous situation. We know, however, that animals exposed to stress for extended periods of time experience chronic cortisol exposures.

The constant release of cortisol is counterproductive to many things, including milk production, fertility, and muscle growth, just to name a few. Side effects from cortisol release may be temporary stresses, such as being sick from disease or being moved to a new group of animals, or may be from a longer-term stress, such as poor feed quality or inadequate housing to protect the animals from the weather elements.

So what do dairy farmers do in order to minimize the stress animals experience on their farms? These are considered best practices:

- Move and work with the animals without using loud voices and noises, stick, electric prods, and anything else the animals may find bothersome.
- Provide an environment where they can be clean and comfortable, have access to fresh, quality feed and water, and where they can interact with their herd mates in a safe manner.
- Treat illnesses in a prompt fashion, including providing for an animal's pain alleviation needs.

I am excited about where the future of animal welfare is going. Not only do we realize alleviating pain is important, but research is expanding in this area. Future medicines will give us more options to effectively manage the pain and discomfort of food-producing animals.

Animal care isn't an afterthought in what we do in agriculture; it's at the forefront of what we do every day. I see farmers on a daily basis that care deeply about their animal care, whether they have a large farm or small farm. It's certainly my top priority as a veterinarian. Just because an animal will end its life as a source of food doesn't mean that it shouldn't be treated humanely while it is alive.

Swift holds herself—and the farmers she works with—accountable to these standards. Veterinarians are a critical part of animal health and welfare on a farm to ensure safe food.

5. Are Confined Spaces Cruel?

ROBOTIC COWS AT THE SCIENCE FAIR

My daughter recently completed her seventh year of science fair. She wanted to include dairy cattle in her science experiment. Every year. As a mom, I love watching her brain light on fire with this hands-on learning, but it can get a bit tense after seven years of helping design an experiment with dairy cattle that an elementary student can do.

> **Food Truth**
>
> Housing is used to protect animals—and your food— from nature.

Last year she looked at the digestibility of six different feeds (soybeans, cottonseed, corn, hay, etc.) while working with a very kind PhD student to use a fistulated cow (the same kind that saved Peppermint's life—one with a surgically placed cannula in her side) at the Purdue University dairy farm. The highlight was when she put her arm inside the research cow's stomach through the fistula and felt the contraction of rumination (how cows digest their food). That was enough to keep her chattering about cow innards for six months!

You can imagine the pressure this year, her last year of science fair. Thankfully, she became fascinated with robots last fall at World Dairy Expo. Expo is similar to fashion week in New York, but for beautiful dairy cows in Madison, Wisconsin. She would stand in rapt attention watching the robotic milkers whenever I had meetings. When it came time to go to another area, she'd tell me about the ways she'd redesign the robots. She left Expo saying that she wanted to use cows and robots for science fair that year.

Friends helped us come up with the idea to compare locomotion (how well a cow moves) with cows milked by robots to those milked in a regular parlor (the location cattle go to be milked). Kuehnert Dairy Farm, two hours east of us, has both a parlor and robots and was gracious enough to work with her in conducting the science fair experiment.

Interestingly, my daughter's science fair results showed that cows being milked by four robots had better locomotion and higher milk production. Technology on the farm isn't only cool—it also can also help animals.

The big questions and food myths:

- *Why would you keep animals in those metal buildings?*
- *Shouldn't all cows be out on pasture?*

CONFINED SPACES AND GREEN PLACES

What is the best housing for cows? It depends on the farm.

Some operations, like the Kuenherts near Fort Wayne, Indiana, have an ultra-modern facility. They have 250 cows milked by robots, plus a few in the parlor. The family—a dad and two brothers with their wives—open their farm doors to host a fall festival attracting over 15,000 visitors.

After hanging out with the cows while my daughter was conducting her experiment, there was no doubt that the cows were happy being milked by robots. It was kind of funny to watch how much cows enjoy robotic milkers; some cows went to the robot to be milked six or seven times each day.

Did you know each milking robot costs around $200,000? Nathan Kuenhert, one of the brothers operating the family farm, points to his cow's health improvements in the 15 months the robots have been a part of the farm. The robots, as compared to the 52-year-old milking parlor, not only improved the cow's quality of life, but did the same for Nathan's family since cows have to be milked 365 days a year.

I can tell you without a doubt these cows were happy. They showed it in a few different ways:

1. The cows were annoyingly friendly—they were happy to wrap our long hair in their tongue while my daughter locomotion-scored about 50 cows. Cattle that are sick prefer to be left alone, so it was clear the cows were healthy.
2. Their body condition, as well as their foot and leg health (a critical measurement of health in dairy cattle), were both excellent. In other words—they were moving well, slept in sand beds (preferred by dairy cows everywhere), and had outstanding nutrition.
3. Their milk production was excellent—and unhappy cows do not produce a lot of milk.

There Are Many Ways to House Dairy Cattle

Some operations will keep their cows out on pasture, like my neighbors, so the cows aren't in the barn a lot during the summer and fall. However, even those cows are in the barn for shelter during weather, to eat their specially mixed ration (a nutritionally balanced feed mix), and to get milked.

WIDESPREAD ABUSE ON DAIRY FARMS?

"Dairy cows being abused" is an increasingly common headline. It's important to remember context, which is tough to do if you have not been on a dairy farm. For example, you may find it disgusting to sleep in a bed of sand, but cows love it. What may be cruel for your dog is not necessarily so for a cow.

Since cows wear their leather coats every day, they can handle a lot of cold, but protecting their udders is a priority. It's especially important in the cold for dairy farmers who live in harsh winters. Those who live in a more arid area are concerned with keeping the udders clean during times of high rain, when it's muddy.

Shelter for milking cows is really important because their teats (each cow has an udder with four teats hanging down) can get frostbitten or damaged in the mud. Frostbitten teats can be permanently damaged, leading to more mastitis (an infection that is hard on the cow and expensive to treat). Mastitis is most commonly treated with antibiotics, but the milk is withheld so it does not enter the food supply.

Likewise, providing shade for cattle not housed in barns in extreme heat is important. Dairies will have shades so that their cattle can better handle the heat. Clean drinking water is always important, but especially critical during periods of high heat. Cows are also monitored for panting; many dairies have overhead sprinklers to keep their cattle cooler.

Other operations have 2,500 cows they milk three times a day. For example, the cows being milked for Fairlife milk are part of an operation that includes tens of thousands of cows. The same is true for some major organic brands. Is large bad? Not necessarily. In fact, the larger the operation, the longer the list of regulations.

Some dairy farmers put cattle out on pasture a good part of the year. New Zealand is known for that because of their climate, but it's also done in the United States. These operations require a lot of pasture management, have reduced feed costs, and typically have a lower milk production. And most farms today have a metal barn with closed doors—not to hide anything, but to protect their animals' biosecurity. These metal barns, while not as pretty as the old wooden barns of yesteryear, are a significant improvement in cow comfort and biosecurity because animals are protected from the elements and diseases from other species.

The view from my office is Holsteins out on grass. It is beautiful, but there are different ways to keep cows happy in both confined spaces and green places. Why does a dairy farmer choose one way over the other? They choose what works for their family, cattle, and resources. The critical factor is being sure the cows are managed well, which includes keeping a close eye on cow comfort, health, and nutrition from the time they are babies.

CARING FOR BABY CALVES

Did you know that the care and housing for calves (baby cows) is a really big deal on a dairy farm?

Bassinets for calves come in a variety of forms, none that look like bassinets from a hospital nursery—but all are calf pens. It's essential for the calf to have fresh air, a dry bed, protection from the elements (along with plenty of nutritious food, of course), and plenty of room to move around. Calf care is a priority on dairy farms, and calves are checked a few times each day.

Calves are often housed in hutches, which look like little white houses. They can also be housed in pens in a greenhouse or hoop barn. They are usually separated so they can't suck on each other (to prevent the spread of illness) until they are over a month old. Some calves are fed with robotic feeders; others are fed in buckets or bottles by a person who specializes in calf care.

As a calf grows older, her diet changes from milk to grain to forage (grass, hay, silage, haylage). Calves are placed in groups—it's similar to an elementary class that goes through school together. They may be in a barn, on pasture, or both. Once they are bred to a bull and then calve at two years of age, they enter the milking herd and are housed with the cows.

Regardless of the age of the dairy animal, the common denominator is that all types of housing require solid management (husbandry) to know what is working best for the herd. It's similar to managing businesses; all are a little different. Each requires knowledge of the manager about how to best care for their people. There is no single answer to what is the best housing for every dairy cow, just as there is no single answer to managing a business. It's about choice and finding the right benchmarks to measure.

6. Is Organic the Utopia?

A SMALL DAIRY FARMER ON ORGANICS AND ANTIBIOTICS

Joanna didn't grow up on a farm, but she knew from spending time with her grandpa that she loved cows. She's a Cornell graduate, works in agricultural financing, and married a dairy farmer, so they're slowly building their herd.

> **Food Truth**
>
> Organic farming is about production methods, not nutritional value.

They're now living in upstate Vermont, milking 60 little brown cows known as Jerseys and a few Holsteins while raising two adorable boys. She also blogs because she believes in dairy farmers—regardless of size or type of farm—and has testified before Congress on behalf of dairy farmers.

"Why do you farm?" I asked her, just as I did every farmer and rancher interviewed for this book.

"We farm because we have a love for the cows and the land, specifically this land that has been in my husband's family for two generations now. We feel honored to have the privilege to produce food—milk, specifically, given its nutritional value. We are also excited to raise our boys in a farming lifestyle—one rooted in the responsibility and rewards that come with caring for the land and environment and other living beings, especially from such an early age."

In Joanna's own words:

> My guess is that as you approach our farm and see our girls grazing our rolling green hills in Northeast Vermont, you would maybe assume we are an organic herd. We are not, and I will get into the why not at the end of this post.

I know there are some people who choose the certified organic label for other items and extend that preference to milk, which is their choice. But in my opinion, I think it's irresponsible to make people feel guilty if they don't want to or can't shell out the extra cash for the label without an adequate explanation, especially when budgets are tight.

When companies sell products, they're obviously looking for an edge. This comes in the form of price or quality, for example, but ultimately their edge is based on consumer perception. Labels and other retail packaging are often used to convey a claim to alter the perception of the product in order to sell more or to sell at a higher price. This often leaves products without special labels looking somehow inferior with no adequate explanation. It underscores the importance for food and nutrition professionals to communicate science-based facts about food.

Joanna brings up interesting points about assumptions of what dairy farms look like, food guilt, and consumer fear of what is in milk. These are the questions I most often hear around organic dairy products.

The big questions and food myths:

- *Is organic milk free of hormones and antibiotics?*
- *Aren't organic dairy products healthier for my family?*

THE DAIRY DILEMMA

The dairy case is huge. You read about claims of happy cows, find low-fat and nonfat products, see bucolic pictures on labels, find hormone claims on labels, read pledges of being pure, hear about antibiotics, and . . . it's overwhelming. That's before you even look at "regular" milk as compared to organic milk. Joanna offers more perspective from a person who milks cows every day:

What does the certified organic label on milk mean and why is it so much more expensive? There is no significant difference in the composition of milk that comes from cows that are raised with organic practices or those that are from conventional farms. The same nutrients and hormones exist in both, both are safe to consume, and BOTH are free from antibiotics. Interesting to note, there is no way to test milk to determine whether it was from an organic farm or a conventional farm—or one that uses rbST or one that does not. Bottom line, milk is milk.

Because of the combination of nine essential nutrients, milk—organic or otherwise—packs a powerful punch for a healthy diet. The USDA and the U.S. National Academy of Sciences define an essential nutrient as a dietary substance required for healthy body functioning. The nine found in milk are calcium, potassium, phosphorus, protein, vitamin D, vitamin A, vitamin B_{12}, riboflavin, and niacin.

Sometimes, there can be a very slight difference in fat and protein levels between organic and conventional milk, but research shows this is thought to have more to do with the cows' diet than any other factor. You might see this same difference in milk amongst different brands or from a local, seasonally grazed herd that may or may not be organic.

When it comes to safety, all milk sold in stores is processed to kill harmful bacteria—either through pasteurization or ultra-high temperature processing. However, milk, along with many other food products, is not a sterile product and thus some tolerance is allowed for bacteria counts. In a study examining the composition of milk from organic and conventional farms, the bacteria counts were lower in conventionally labeled milk. However, the difference was minimal, and both were far below the federal limit.

Along those same lines, hormones are present in all milk—organic, rbST-free, conventional, chocolate, strawberry, coffee, skim, 2 percent, etc. The same study found a few small differences in hormone levels between conventional and organic milk. While organic milk was slightly lower in IGF-1, it had higher progesterone and estrogen concentrations than conventional milk. However, these differences are not significant in humans consuming organic or conventional milk.

Finally to be absolutely clear, ALL milk on the shelf in the grocery store is free of antibiotics. Taking it a step further, organic farmers pledge not to use antibiotics on their cattle. If they do, the cow must leave the herd. On a conventional farm, the farmer is allowed to use antibiotics to treat a sick cow. However, the milk she produces is withheld from mixing with the rest of the herd's until it is tested and shown to be clear of the antibiotic. Many tests are done on the milk in its journey from farm to store shelf to ensure that there are no antibiotics present. The farmer risks losing his/her license to sell milk if antibiotics are found.

Regardless of the label claims, this is an area dairy farmers take very seriously.

WHAT IS ORGANIC?

"Organic is a labeling term that indicates that the food or other agricultural product has been produced through approved methods. The organic standards describe the specific requirements that must be verified by a USDA-accredited certifying agent before products can be labeled USDA organic," according to the USDA Web site.[13]

"Organic animal health, like organic crop health, relies on preventative practices and systems. Good genetics are important, as organic livestock producers should select breeds that are well adapted to their particular environment. Balanced nutrition, exercise, and a low-stress environment also contribute to building strong immune systems in animals. Vaccination and other preventative measures are common; antibiotics and growth hormones are prohibited. Organic livestock producers work to manage exposure to disease and parasites through grazing management, proper sanitation, and preventing the introduction of disease agents.

"Organic livestock must eat certified organic feed. Organic feed must be grown and processed by certified organic operations. Similarly, any pastures, forages, and plant-based bedding (such as hay) accessible to livestock must be certified as organically grown and processed. Certain additives, such as vitamins and minerals not produced organically, can be fed to organic livestock in trace amounts."

In regard to genetically modified organisms, the USDA says, "The use of genetic engineering, or genetically modified organisms (GMOs), is prohibited in organic products. This means an organic farmer can't plant GMO seeds, an organic cow can't eat GMO alfalfa or corn, and an organic soup producer can't use any GMO ingredients."[14]

It's important to note all types of dairy farms (conventional and organic) rely on good genetics, balanced nutrition, exercise, vaccination, and low stress levels for the cows. None of those are unique to one production system—those are the basic tenets of caring for dairy cattle. The most significant differences between "regular" and organic dairy farms are in feed types and the ability to treat an animal with medications.

FROM THE MOUTH OF A DAIRY GODDESS

Barbara Martin is a proud grandma, mom, wife, and dairy farmer and branded herself as the Dairy Goddess in 2010. She has a personality as big as California, where she resides in Hanford, near the center of the state. She and her husband milk about 150 cows and farm 120 acres of almonds and alfalfa right along a major highway. They are in the process of transitioning from being a conventional dairy farm to becoming organic.

When I asked her why she started Dairy Goddess, she responded, "We had just gotten over the worst financial disasters for the dairy industry in 2009. In California, from 2009 to 2012 the state has lost 500 dairy farms with many more still exiting. We knew we had to do something different if we wanted to remain in the dairy business. We saw the trend of consumers wanting to know where their food comes from and supporting local farmers."

Barbara and I got to know each other because of social media back in 2009. Her love for her animals was clear, as she would often post pictures of what her favorite cow was doing. Barbara is quick to help anything that would connect farmers with food buyers—regardless of what type of farm it is.

"I worked with other farmers in social media telling our story so I decided that creating a product on the farm would be a great way to keep the conversation going as well as creating a value-added product from our farm." And that she has! It's been fun watching her build her very first room with dairy processing to her travels to various food shows and farmers' markets throughout California to the advent of their own farm stand.

Since I lived in Barbara's area for a few years early in my career, I'm familiar with the dairy scene there and had to ask, "Why are you transitioning to organic?"

Having a granddaughter now and our world just moving so quickly and everything becoming so large we decided as a family that we wanted to slow down a bit and to show my grandchildren, as well as others, a bit of the organic practices that our grandparents showed and passed down to us. We have gotten older. We are tired of dealing with so many employees and the search for good quality employees. We grew tired of California's harsh environmental regulations along with California's drought and fight/expense for water.

It was a difficult decision for us as we had always farmed progressively. The hardest part is that when you have a sick animal you are not able to treat them with antibiotics and keep them within your herd. So we are working with our neighbors to take those animals in case they need to be treated. Though working with a small herd we are able to be proactive and treat the animals with more homeopathic remedies.

Does she believe having "organic" on her products makes them more valuable?

"Many people support organic and organic farming practices. Those people are willing to spend more for those practices. With my market and the Dairy Goddess niche, my customers appreciate organic practices. They always want to know about our farm and show such interest in coming to see our farm. We live off of a major highway. We decided to open a farm stand to sell our products as a way to continue to tell our story and show them firsthand."

Dairy Goddess is known for fresh cheeses and curds, but also bottles nonhomogenized-vat pasteurized whole milk and whole chocolate milk. It is a family operation; Barbara's daughter manages the production of dairy products and coordinates markets and deliveries. Barbara handles all sales, marketing, and promotion. Her husband runs all of the farming and dairy.

"We, of course, all work together and help wherever we are needed at whatever needs to be done. Our cows are our number one priority, just as they always have been. Not only are they our livelihood, but we believe our gifts that God has entrusted them to us and have a moral obligation to their care and well being. That was true when we were 'conventional' and is still true as we transition to organic."

I asked, "What has been the most difficult challenge in the change from conventional to organic?"

"The paperwork and adjusting to all of the requirements required by organic regulations. Paperwork and keeping good records. There is a lot to do and learn, but we are excited for this next part of our journey. Oh, one more thing, the extra weeds take some getting used to, too (laughing)."

WHERE DID THE ORGANIC LABEL COME FROM?

The 1990 National Organic Food Production Act directed the USDA to establish (1) a national organic production certification program, (2) a label for organically produced agricultural products, (3) a national list of approved and prohibited substances to be included in the organic production standards, and (4) an accreditation program for agents who would certify conformance. The act was a reaction to a need to standardize the organic label.[15]

Two skeptics of the organic label said in a *Forbes* article, "The meaning of the USDA organic label was muddled from the beginning. By creating this marketing tool, USDA conferred a valuable seal of approval on products made by

USDA-certified producers with government-sanctioned processes and procedures that are in no way related to safety, nutrition or quality."

They went on to point at the release of the final national organic standards.
Then Secretary of Agriculture Dan Glickman said, "Let me be clear about one
thing, the organic label is a marketing tool. It is not a statement about food safety.
Nor is 'organic' a value judgment about nutrition or quality."[15]

You decide. Is organic worth the extra money? I absolutely support farm families like Barbara's for their right to farm organically—and capture a niche market. However, it saddens me when a mother chooses soda over milk because she
can't afford $8 for a gallon of organic milk. Studies show slight differences in both
organic and conventional exist, but there is not a clear nutritional advantage of
any production type. A $4 gallon of milk has just as much nutrition as that $8
gallon of milk.

IS THE RIGHT BRAND BIG BUSINESS OR SMALL BUSINESS?

Many believe they are supporting small business owners like Barbara when they
buy organic. However, there is another side to organic—big business. While
organics still only account for 4 percent of annual food sales, it is a $32 billion
market annually. Many larger food companies, such as General Mills, Coca-Cola,
and Kellogg have bought out organic businesses to tap into those sales.

"Some of these big companies go out of their way to hide their ties to the organic
labels," said Phil Howard, an associate professor at Michigan State University, who
has tracked the changes and provided them to the *Washington Post*. "They know
that consumers tend to be skeptical of the corporations, that a person who buys
organic is often someone looking for an alternative to conventional food."[16]

What matters most? The "right" label from the "right" brand or the right nutrition? Nutrition is always the most important—your family getting dairy servings
in as a part of a balanced diet. Know milk is produced with consistent standards,
whether it came from a farm with 200 cows or 2,000 cows—regular or organic.
Both types of milk are produced from farms whose owners do their best to take
care of their cows.

Milk is a nutritional powerhouse—regardless of whether it came from an
organic farm or a conventional operation. Organic farming is about a style of production, not nutritional value.

Table 1   Dairy Case Food Truths

Food Myth	Food Truth
Hormones are bad.	**Food Truth 1: Hormones are in everything.** Hormones are the chemical messenger of life. They are in every product, including plant-based foods.
Antibiotics are in milk.	**Food Truth 2: Antibiotics have benefits.** Your dairy products do not contain antibiotic residues. All USDA Grade A milk is tested extensively to ensure this. Whether milk or cottage cheese, antibiotics are not allowed!
Dairy cattle are abused.	**Food Truth 3: Animal welfare is an hourly concern on farms and ranches.** Unhappy cows don't make milk. Farmers don't become dairy farmers unless they like cows; dairy cattle require care 24/7.
Cows in barns are unhappy.	**Food Truth 4: Housing is used to protect animals—and your food—from nature.** A balanced diet, clean bed, and getting milked regularly keeps cows happy—and your milk healthy.
Organic is always the most nutritious and ethical choice.	**Food Truth 5: Organic farming is about production methods, not nutritional value.** Milk, organic or not, is a nutritious and necessary part of your diet—regardless of how it was produced.

Part II: Eggs

How many choices can fit in one small space? Thirty-six different types of egg label claims in a less-than-10-foot area point out the overwhelming nature of eggs; this will help guide you to finding the right egg for your family in spite of the guilt-laden labels.

"Thinking is difficult, that's why people judge."

—Carl Jung

7. Animal Care, in Context

PUPPY LOVE IN THE PASTURE

Every morning and evening, I'm greeted by 250 pounds of love. This affection comes whether it's hot or cold, dusk or dawn, in snow drifts or sauna-like temperatures. The love bounds up to the wood gate behind my barn and unabashedly throws paws bigger than my fists up on top of the gate, looking for a hug. Big brown eyes look at me with pure trust and joy. But then there is the drool . . . gobs of drool dripping down my arm, leg, or business clothes.

> **Food Truth**
>
> Housing is used to protect animals—and your food— from nature.

If you've ever known a Great Pyrenees, you can appreciate what it's like to be loved by two puppies, each growing to 125 pounds of stubbornly independent intelligence. The brother and sister, Astro and Sugar, are intensely loyal to our family, even when it's overwhelming—or the gate breaks under their enthusiasm. I'm fairly certain they would follow my daughter over burning coals and know that they will go through a fence for her.

They also watch over our livestock, keeping the coyotes away from calves and monitoring the pasture for wildlife like skunks. The dogs' love for cattle runs deep enough that they enjoy daily baths from sandpapery cow tongues.

But as much as I love them, I know these beautiful dogs are not human, not my children. They are pets and do not have human needs, nor do they have human intellect.

The big questions and food myths:

- *Is it wrong for chickens to be in cages?*
- *Isn't it more natural for birds to roam?*

ANIMALS ARE NOT HUMANS

In a society where we embrace rodents as cartoon characters, give pigs a political voice, and fill advertisements with grinning cows, we seem to forget that animals do not have the same intelligence or abilities as humans. Animals' lives deserve to be respected and valued—but they are not humans.

As such, animals have different housing needs. For example, I was feeling really guilty the dogs couldn't get inside during a particularly nasty January snowstorm, and that guilt overcame my ability to think. The wind chill was near zero, large quantities of snow were falling, and it was miserable to be outside. My worry was being fed by messages on Facebook about how important it is to bring your pets in during bad weather.

When I went out in the driving wind and snow to check on Astro and Sugar, intending to let them in the barn, I found them wrestling in the pasture as winter blew all around them. They were playing in the snow with joy! You see, Pyrenees were bred in the mountains of France. They were bred for cold weather. And they were perfectly happy with being outside in the snow and wind, even though it may seem cruel if you are not familiar with their breeding.

The same is true for farm animals; housing may seem cruel if taken out of context. Farmers know their animals firsthand, have studied the species' breeding, understand the animal's instincts, and work hard to provide the best conditions for a given animal.

For example, consider chickens. Isn't it more natural for Henny Penny to be outside, pecking corn off the ground? It's also natural for Henny Penny to freeze to death, eat trash, be killed by predators, and poop on her egg (increasing your risk for salmonella). And if Henny Penny gets mad or her fellow chicken is ill, she may decide to peck the other chicken to death.

As a result, most chickens live in a temperature-controlled barn in some sort of cage. Their eggs immediately leave the cage so there is little exposure to bacteria from manure. Today's laying hens have constant access to food and water 24 hours a day, oblivious to the drama that surrounds them about housing. Critically thinking about housing instead of marketing labels would increase logic in the egg case and decrease food drama.

IS IT A FACTORY FARM IF CHICKENS ARE IN CAGES?

Dianne McComb is an egg farmer just north of London, Ontario, in Canada (north of Ohio). She's passionate about eggs and chickens and also has experience with beef cattle, corn, wheat, and soybeans.

"Farming is an equal opportunity business for women. Scraping manure is a non-gender job. Gathering eggs is good for all ages and walking rows is good exercise for a gal after too many meetings," she says.

"What's the history of the farm's laying hens?" I asked her, as I was curious what it was like in Canada.

"In 1962 we built our first hen barn to house 2,000 laying hens. The hens were raised from chicks to pullets by us and the eggs were 2/3 for delivery into London restaurants and homes, while the other 1/3 was shipped to a grading station. The hens in the new barn were placed in cages as opposed to the hens running in large rooms upstairs on the second level of the banked barn (a traditional wood barn).

In those days, the hens laid about 220 eggs per hen and the mortality was as high as 10 percent, but that was an improvement over the bank barn results."

"It's amazing to think about 2,000 hens way back in 1962," I said. "So how has your farm changed?"

"Today, with the addition of a second barn and new conventional housing, allowing the hens more space, we have quota for 26,000 hens. We are full to the space requirement allowed by the Egg Board.

"Our little hens are amazing! Although they look no different from their ancestors, they now lay 330 eggs annually and have less than a 1.5 percent mortality rate. They have different nutritional requirements (still basic corn, wheat, soymeal with vitamins/minerals balance), but eat less and are less aggressive. The breed I have is called a Shaver."

I asked her about birds in cages, what she sees firsthand, and the potential impact on food safety.

"When the birds had the run of the upstairs of the barn, there was a high loss of hens and eggs due to disease, rodents, contact with feces, cannibalism of hens, and eggs that were cracked or too dirty.

"We changed to house hens in cages to improve their lives and eggs safety as neither hen nor egg was in contact with manure. Those conventional units (cages) have changed to include more space for the hen to eat, drink and rest."

But how does she know cages are the right thing for her animals?

Dianne's passion for her hens becomes apparent as she explains:

"When I walk into the hen house I hear a sound of hens not stressed, they're communicating with others in the barn. If I were to clap my hands they will all stop to see what the different noise is then start up again when they are sure all is good. It is no different walking the rows of my barn looking into the eyes of my many hens than looking at any other living creature.

"My chickens need me to be sure they have the correct feed for their stage of development, the fresh and available water, and that the air is moving by their unit. Walking by I check for any birds that are ill or deceased and remove them respectfully as they have served me and my family.

"This is not a factory. This is my family farm and I care for my hens to provide a safe product for consumers. These cages do not harm the hens. There are pluses and minuses to any style of housing, but it's hard for people to understand them if they have not worked with laying hens."

Dianne knows that there is constant change in farming in both the United States and Canada. She points to the most recent study by the Coalition for Sustainable Egg Supply, comparing the different housing types. "As egg farmers, we are standing up for the welfare of the hen and promoting the enriched colony or furnished colony. It allows the hen the ability to display many of her natural instincts like nesting in privacy, perching, scratching, and grouping to eat. Each colony can hold between 30 and 50 birds, and eggs do not come in contact with the manure as they gently roll onto the belt which moves them to the gathering area for daily collection and twice weekly pick up."

ARE YOU BEING MISLED ABOUT YOUR EGGS?

Just as there are many different styles of schools today, from Montessori to public school to co-op to homeschool, there are many different ways to house chickens. Those who have firsthand familiarity with the situation are best equipped to make that decision.

Letting hens out of cages sounds rational. It seems like logical animal welfare. But it fails to address what science says is best and ignores common sense from people like Dianne who care for hens every day.

There's more than one way to raise a hen, but keep in mind, a sick or unhappy chicken does not produce eggs. That's the practical tip from the farm you can keep in the back of your mind as a comfort about animal welfare when you buy eggs. Chickens have to be happy and healthy to produce eggs—regardless of the way they are raised—or you wouldn't have those tasty eggs in your grocery cart.

Instead, there is a history of animal rights groups influencing food buyers through "pressure campaigns." They put restaurants, brands, and food retailers in the spotlight with misleading messages about company XYZ being supportive of the mistreatment of animals. Companies bend to the pressure, wishing to protect their sales and reputation.

Rather than bending to activist pressure, wouldn't it make more sense to look at the scientific measures around what is best for a chicken, coupled with input from those who are most familiar with laying hens? A rational approach seems a lot more reasonable than being misled in the egg case.

I buy conventionally raised eggs and shop on price because I trust the system in place—and that egg farmers like Dianne know the best care for the birds.

8. Pecking Order Isn't Pretty

CHICKENS AS BULLIES

Remember your days in junior high and high school? Finding your place in the different groups? Navigating cliques? Knowing where to sit in the lunch room? I recall moving to a new school in seventh grade. The pecking order and trying to find my place was, by far, the hardest adjustment. Seventh and eighth grade girls can be some of the meanest creatures on earth—very much like chickens pecking at each other. And if you're not aware, chickens do bully.

> **Food Truth**
> Animal welfare is an hourly concern on farms and ranches.

The big questions and food myths:

- *Why would you do some of those practices to those cute little chicks?*
- *Are chickens pumped full of hormones and antibiotics?*

THE CRUELNESS OF PECKING ORDERS

Warning—you may change the way you look at animals. You see, chickens are cannibals. They will peck and peck at each other until . . . well, you know. They are also among the world's largest scavenger population. Chickens don't just wait for a farmer to thrown corn down and happily peck the ground. They will eat what they find. Corn. Bugs. Feces. Garbage. Oats. Worms. Each other.

Wait . . . what? Yes, I said chickens will eat each other. Chickens are omnivores, which means they eat both plants and animals. They will injure one other, bully a weaker chicken, and eat a sick bird. Animals naturally operate in a hierarchy that ensures survival of the fittest. Although it may seem gross to you, animals follow this hierarchy even when that doesn't fit into idyllic images of farms.

Before you get too grossed out and never eat an egg again, let me explain why I'm sharing this. It's important to understand animal behavior—even when it is gross—if you're going to judge animal welfare. That's called full transparency, and it's not always pretty. The American Veterinary Medical Association defines animal welfare as "the state of the animal; the treatment that an animal receives is covered by other terms such as animal care, animal husbandry and humane treatment."

It is a farmer's job to protect the state of the animal, in concert with professionals like veterinarians. It is not a simple task; there are actually college degrees and academia that focus exclusively on the care of poultry. Protecting the state of the animal involves science, patience, the ability to read animals, and protocols.

One way farmers protect chickens from each other is by beak management. This technique, similar to trimming toenails, keeps the beak blunt so they can't peck each other. Is it cruel? Not unless you consider trimming your nails cruel.

However, taken out of context, with no knowledge of what animals can do to each other—a video or photo of a chick having its beak trimmed can look awful. Pause when you see these images and think about context. Why would a farmer use that practice with animals? What is the consequence if they don't?

Today's chicken farms are highly regulated; most chickens live in a temperature-controlled barn so they are not out in the heat or snow. They have access to food and water 24 hours a day. They have a belt that takes away their manure. And contrary to some claims, laying hens are not fed growth promotants or antibiotics. It's illegal to do so.

However, hens are vaccinated for salmonella through their breast bone, which has been attributed to improving food safety. Cages have also prevented diseases from spreading since they have limited exposure to other birds. And healthy hens lay the best eggs.

WHAT DOES FREEDOM MEAN TO A CHICKEN?

The Coalition for Sustainable Egg Supply (www.sustainableeggcoaliton.org) brings together the experts and science of laying hens (which are different from chickens used for meat). The group conducted a study with scientists from Michigan State University; University of California, Davis; Iowa State University; and USDA Agricultural Research Service.[17]

They studied the positive and negative impacts of the three different types of housing systems for laying hens. All are indoors, have constant access to food and water, and have a belt manure management system to keep the manure away from the birds.

1. Conventional cage: Hens are housed in cages with wire mesh floors.
2. Enriched colony: Hens are housed in colonies of about 60 birds in multilevel rows of enclosures with wire mesh floors. Access is given for specific bird behaviors such as scratching, perching, nesting, and dust bathing.
3. Cage-free aviary: Hens are able to move about specific sections of the barn and have access to multiple levels so they can perch, dust bathe, scratch, and nest. A typical aviary section holds 1,660 birds.

The study looked at a lot of different factors related to sustainability, but the findings related to animal health and welfare were the same as what Dianne shared from her experience on the farm.

"Hen mortality was much higher in the aviary system due to a variety of conditions, including hypocalcemia, egg yolk peritonitis, and to behavioral issues, with hens either being excessively pecked, or picked out (vent). There was less mortality in the enriched colony due to behavioral issues, and the least in the conventional system. There was the most egg yolk peritonitis in the conventional cages, less in the aviary and the least in the enriched colony. It was also harder to detect dead birds in the aviary and enriched colonies than in conventional cages."

In other words, taking hens out of cages isn't necessarily the kindest system. Cage-free eggs are not the only answer! The research shows that the three different housing systems all have pros and cons. There is no one system that is definitively better for hens on all counts.

9. Eggstravaganza or Overwhelmed?

FEELING OVERWHELMED IN THE EGG CASE

At least once a year, one of my self-proclaimed nerd friends and I take a "field trip" to a new grocery store. Jennie has a PhD in meat science and analyzes food buying in painful detail, so it's always an entertaining experience. Two years ago, I took her to one of my favorite stores from my California days, Trader Joe's, who had recently moved into the Indianapolis area and do a decent job of offering choice between traditional food products, organics, and niche items.

> **Food Truth**
> Marketing on labels is confusing consumers.

We smiled at the lovely flowers, meandered through the international cheese and specialty meats case with thoughts of serving delightful appetizers to our friends. We were happily watching food buyers and getting a foodie fix. Then we happened upon the egg case. And my head started spinning.

In a small area, roughly $4' \times 8'$, there were over a dozen different types of labels. Generic, organic, cage free, vegan raised, brown, omega-fed, natural, free range, antibiotic free, white, purple with green stripes, etc. I'll say it again; a dozen different labels in about a 32-square-foot area. Talk about being overwhelmed in the egg case!

How did this hyperbole get out of control? Marketing. I don't know if marketing departments operate under the philosophy of "confuse them and charge them a premium"—but it sure seems like it with some food products. Let's take a look at learning how to simplify buying eggs.

The big questions and food myths:

- *What do I really need to know to make the right choice for my family?*
- *Why are there so many choices?*

DID THE CHICKEN, THE EGG, OR THE LABEL COME FIRST?

I believe in choice—both on the farm and the plate. However, choice created by marketing claims creates confusion. I can only imagine the confusion people have about eggs; I know the difference in the label claims and could barely get through the egg case.

Perhaps this is too simple, but at the grocery store I buy white eggs from chickens grown in cages and fed regular diets. I do not pander to brand claims; I shop on price and typically choose white eggs without cracks that are furthest from their expiration date. Why?

One, because it's simple. Who has time to be perusing a dozen egg choices and analyzing the merits of each label claim?

Second, because I know and trust the system put in place by USDA and Food and Drug Administration (FDA). The FDA is an agency within the U.S. Department of Health and Human Services, dating back to the Pure Food and Drugs Act passed in 1906. The FDA is responsible for protecting the public health by assuring the safety, efficacy, and security of human and veterinary drugs, biological products, medical devices, our nation's food supply, cosmetics, and products that emit radiation.[18]

"The United States Department of Agriculture (USDA) works to support the American agricultural economy to strengthen rural communities; to protect and conserve our natural resources; and to provide a safe, sufficient, and nutritious food supply for the American people. The Department's wide range of programs and responsibilities touches the lives of every American every day."[19]

You may not share trust in the government agencies regulating our food supply, but given the strict guidelines in place for the chickens that produce these eggs and then the processing before eggs get to the store, it's worthy of your exploration.

By the way, I also buy eggs from our neighbors. Brown eggs from free-range chickens. Not because they're necessarily a better choice, but because I like to support our neighbor and am often out of time, so I can run down there 40 minutes faster than I can get to the closest grocery store and back home. It is possible to make different choices for your family, depending on the pressures of the day.

There is no nutritional difference between a brown egg and a white egg; the eggs just come from different breeds of chickens. A brown egg comes from a hen with red feathers and brownish-red ear lobes, whereas a white egg is from a hen with white feathers and white ear lobes. Neither is a more superior breed.

AN EGG IS AN EGG, REGARDLESS OF LABEL CLAIMS

An egg is an egg is an egg. The nutritional value is somewhat based upon what a laying hen is fed, but unless you have a specific dietary need, grab your carton of eggs and go.

Laying hens in cages eat a balanced corn-based ration, including soybean meal, wheat, sorghum, barley, and oats. Their ration is likely to include supplemental vitamins and minerals and may include meat meal for added protein or bone meal for added calcium. Because chickens are omnivores, they naturally eat meat, bones, and grains, which always makes me wonder why it's so awful to supplement meat or bone meal eat in their diet. Frankly, it's unnatural for hens to not have these sources of protein or calcium. The use of these products as feed also means there is natural recycling happening, as the products would end up in a landfill if not consumed. There is a science in balancing a diet for nutrition and taste so the chickens produce the healthiest egg possible.

Hens have the luxury of living in a temperature-controlled barn and have access to water 24/7. Yes, the majority of egg-producing chickens live in cages, as it keeps the price of your eggs down and protects chickens from each other. A lot of work has been done around animal care, but their welfare is monitored closely. Keep in mind that unhappy and unhealthy chickens quit laying eggs.

Chickens are scavengers, which means that free-range chickens will happily eat anything they can dig up, including worms, their own feces, trash, and huge bugs. As one of my chicken-raising friends says, "They're the dumpster divers of the poultry world." I'm not against free-range chickens, but the reality is that chickens, left to their own devices, are scavengers and they can carry the diseases that go along with being a scavenger.

Backyard chickens have become quite trendy, which is a great way for people to experience farm animals. Yet, backyard chickens also come with risks of disease, salmonella, and other concerns. If you have chickens, be sure that everyone—especially children—wash their hands when handling the chickens or eggs to reduce the risk of salmonella.

Luckily, today's modern egg production techniques include rolling belts that immediately remove the eggs so they stay clean (and are fresher). Each egg is gently washed and immediately packed, then sent to the grocery store. It's an amazingly efficient process.

You can verify how old the eggs are yourself. All cartons of USDA Grade A eggs show the packing date and processing plant number, plus it may contain the sell by date. Look at the end of the carton. There will be a P number, which is the processing plant number. The packing date is next, but the secret to this is that it's a Julian date. For example, January 1 is 001 and December 31 is 365 (representing consecutive days of the year), according to Alice Heinemann, MS, RDN, and Joyce Jensen, REHS, CFSP.[20]

Did you know you can store eggs three to five weeks beyond the packing date? Some states do not allow the use of a "sell-by date," so this quick tip can alleviate some concerns around egg expiration.

If you're still concerned about the age of your egg, you can always do a float test. Carefully lower an egg into a bowl of water; if it floats, discard it. If it doesn't, the egg is good to eat. If it floats, that means there's been enough time for air to enter the egg, which helps the egg become buoyant.

Once you get through finding and understanding the expiration date, don't stress about the rest of the claims on your dozen of eggs. Here's a quick breakdown of label claims to save you some time when you buy eggs.

- *Hormone-free:* One of the most misleading, as all eggs contain hormones and no laying hens are allowed to be given hormones.
- *Antibiotic-free:* Another marketing claim. All eggs in the United States are antibiotic free. Any eggs produced by hens being treated with antibiotics for illness would not be sold for human consumption, per FDA regulations.
- *Omega-3 supplemented:* Because eggs are not a significant source of omega-3s, you'd have to eat six or seven eggs in order to meet the suggested daily requirement. Instead, try a tablespoon of soybean or canola oil, or a handful of walnuts.

- *Vegetarian:* Hens are fed only plant-based diets, most likely corn fortified with amino acids since chickens are naturally omnivores. In other words, they're happiest eating grain and bugs and other meat.
- *Farm fresh:* A feel-good claim, but eggs in all modern systems are moved from the hen to processing to packing to the grocery store as fast as possible—therefore, all eggs are farm fresh.
- *Organic:* Certified organic eggs must be verified by a third party, as mandated by USDA organic standards. They have to be cage free and fed an organic diet without any animal protein. Wonder what happens if the hen grabs a worm or catches a bug in this scenario? These birds have to be cage free and have access to the outdoors, although this remains undefined. No hormones are allowed, which is the same as all poultry production, and antibiotics are prohibited (which can lead to animal welfare concerns).
- *Housing (cage free, conventional, pasture, free-range):* The most common types of housing were defined in Chapter 9. Keep in mind that free-range and pasture raised do not necessarily mean that the hen is wandering happily around a luxurious green pasture, and a cage for a chicken is not the same as a cage for your dog.
- *Natural:* What egg isn't natural? Natural is an overused, unregulated term. Natural+Label=Marketing.
- *Brown vs. white:* Genetics in action, with no nutritional differences. Brown eggs typically are more expensive because the hens laying them are larger and require more feed.
- *Certified:* There is a bevy of certification programs to try to "help" food buyers, but the number of certifiers has created more confusion than clarity. I believe the USDA and FDA have the best standards out there.

The majority of consumers buy classic white eggs. As one chicken farmer told me, "It's best for the hens (based upon science), has the lowest carbon footprint, offers the lowest environmental impact and is the most economical."

There is a chain of custody when it comes to food regulations. Mechanisms are put in place by the USDA and FDA, along with the EPA. Prior to believing marketing claims, check this chain of custody. If you are really concerned about an issue, get firsthand information from the people involved. Go back to the actual study instead of the media claim.

Worry about checking the eggs for cracks and the expiration date, and move on. Eat eggs—not marketing.

10. Farmers Buy Food, Too

WHERE DOES YOUR FOOD DOLLAR GO?

Ninety-two percent of Americans consider it "somewhat important" to "very important" that food be affordable, followed by the 91 percent who felt the same way about nutrition, according to the Science and Food Survey released October 2015 by the Chicago Council on Global Affairs.[21]

> **Food Truth**
> Food costs are a shared concern.

Nearly every food survey I've seen over the course of my speaking and writing career lists the price of food in the top three priorities. Farmers and ranchers have worked for decades to keep food costs low by increasing productivity. Some consumers question at what cost, but that sentiment changes as the income bracket goes down.

Americans spend only about 10 percent of their incomes on food, which means our food costs less than anywhere in the world! However, there is a trend toward social issues overcoming efficiency. There are unintended consequences of socially driven decisions ricocheting across our food system. It can create a divide between the food buyer and the food producer, who makes science-driven decisions.

Today farmers receive 16 cents for every dollar you spend on food. You buy $10 worth of eggs and milk, and farmers receive $1.60 of that. Does that seem equitable? Off-farm costs (marketing expenses associated with processing, wholesaling, distributing, and retailing of food products) account for 84 cents of every retail dollar.

In 1980 farmers and ranchers received 31 cents out of every retail dollar spent on food in America. In three decades, the amount farmers received from your food dollar was nearly cut in half. These margins are tough for any business to survive—and the reason why farms have gotten larger.

If you are concerned about food costs, please know that is a shared concern with farmers and ranchers. The people who are raising your food are in the position of being price-takers rather than price-makers.

The big questions and food myths:

- *Why is the price of eggs going up?*
- *Are farmers getting rich?*

THE COST OF DISEASE

Wondering why eggs have cost you more in recent years? Average prices for Grade A large eggs delivered to a Midwest store were around $2.75/dozen in August 2015, which was the most expensive price for a dozen eggs ever seen in this part of the United States. Prices for the same eggs in the same area were about $1.06/dozen in the beginning of 2015.[22]

How do egg prices increase 250 percent in eight months? Goldman Sachs estimated consumers would pay 75 percent more for eggs in 2015, in total $7.5 to $8 billion more across the year.

When laying hens get sick and farmers have to destroy their entire flock, the supply of eggs drops dramatically and cannot keep up with demand, resulting in a rise in price at the grocery store. Avian influenza caused 48 million fowl to die in the first half of 2015—the worst bird flu outbreak in history, according to the USDA. This is not a disease humans can get, nor does it get in your food; the particular strain that destroyed so many birds in 2015 is a virus.

It was spread by migratory birds, and because it is both airborne and spread through the droppings of the wild birds, it is nearly impossible to contain. Contrary to some complaints, avian influenza was not caused by chickens in confined operations. Quite the contrary—"free" birds spread the disease, including backyard chickens. The virus travels in a variety of ways, but the pattern makes it clear that it is not an issue caused by "factory farms."

If you found it painful in the grocery store, imagine the financial impact on the farms that had to put down their entire flock. Hundreds of thousands of dollars in loss, the pain of seeing their animals dead, and great fear for the future.

THE COST OF LEGISLATION

On the West Coast, California is facing its own challenges with eggs, thanks to the passing of Proposition 2. Farmers were required to nearly double the space for each chicken and given seven years to fully come into compliance after the HSUS-pushed legislation. How much did the retrofit cost? $400 million in California alone. And any shell eggs coming into the state—about 30 percent of California's egg supply—must be produced under the same rules. The end result in the grocery store? Eggs priced 35 percent higher than a year prior.[23]

Iowa State University's Egg Industry Center estimates that California will lose 2 to 3 million laying hens because of the space requirements required by the new law. More space per chicken means fewer fowl. "A three percent decrease in egg supply would represent approximately 304 million fewer eggs available in California," concludes research compiled by Maro Ibarburu, an associate scientist and business analyst at Iowa State.

Ibarburu says shopping statistics indicate that each person consumes 15 dozen eggs a year. He estimates that given the reduction in supply and the increase in price, consumers will spend $3.98 more a year on eggs. "This increase would be considered rather modest relative to total food costs," he writes in his report.[24]

THE COST OF CHANGING HOUSING

The Coalition for Sustainable Egg Supply study that included two flocks of hens over a three-year period, comparing hens in conventional, enriched colony, and cage-free hen housing, told a story of change in food costs. All of the costs from this study are listed per dozen of eggs in comparison to a conventional cage system, the current standard for laying hens.

The aviary system had the highest costs, by far.

- Total capital costs 179 percent higher
- Operating costs 23 percent higher
- Total costs 36 percent higher
- Higher feed costs due to decreased production per hen
- Highest labor costs of all systems

The enriched colony system also had higher costs, though not quite as extreme.

- Total capital costs 106 percent higher
- Operating costs 4 percent higher
- Total costs 13 percent higher
- Higher routine labor weekly costs, but reduced overall

There is a ripple effect of unintended consequences across the grocery store when people are making rules or wanting change when they don't understand the business. Price is one of those ripple effects. Farmers are not getting rich; they are facing higher production costs with lower profit margin. Where is the extra margin going? Regulations cost. Legislation costs. Changing housing costs. Diseases cost. Marketing labels cost. All of which add up to more expensive food for all of us.

Table 2   Egg Case Food Truths

Food Myth	Food Truth
It is wrong for a chicken to be in a cage.	**Food Truth 4: Housing is used to protect animals—and your food—from nature.** Chickens are both cannibals and scavengers. They are also hunted by other species. Housing makes for safer food.
Chickens are abused.	**Food Truth 3: Animal welfare is an hourly concern on farms and ranches.** Chickens of today live in regulated temperatures, have fresh water, food to meet their every need, and caretakers who constantly check them.
Labels explain how my eggs were produced.	**Food Truth 6: Marketing on labels is confusing consumers.** Just because a claim is on a label, one product is not superior or inferior to another.
Farmers are profiting from the rise in egg prices.	**Food Truth 7: Food costs are a shared concern.** Increased regulations have led to significantly higher costs and more challenges in egg production.

Part III: Fruits

We love our bananas for breakfast and strawberries in December and then demand locally grown fruit. A realistic look at food miles, worms in fruits, food safety, and our demands for the utopia of perfect fruit that is chemical free. There's more science than you know in the fruit case!

"*Great ideas often receive violent opposition from mediocre minds.*"

—Albert Einstein

11. Is Your Fruit Creating an Environmental Frenzy?

SATURDAY MORNINGS AT THE FARMERS' MARKET

One summer, in the early days of my speaking business, I was a vendor at the biggest farmers' market in my county. Each Saturday morning, my loaves of French bread were such a hit that I finally quadrupled the price so they didn't sell out in the first hour, even after I started offering focaccia bread. I also put together beautiful bouquets of flowers from my wildflower patch and sold a few vegetables that seemed "pretty" enough.

> **Food Truth**
>
> Local is not always better for the environment.

"Are these organic?" "How did you make or grow these?" The questions were always about the source (my garden and kitchen) and the way they were produced. That was 15 years ago—and those two questions likely remain the driving query behind farmers' markets. It just seems better to talk to your farmer, to know the food was raised in your area, and to shake hands with those who produced it, right?

At the risk of completely ruining the farmers market experience, are you sure the food is from your area? I've seen people selling peaches in Wisconsin in June, which most certainly are not local (and likely shipped in from several states away), regardless of the label placed on the crate. I can also tell you that I know vendors who sell their produce as organic after they go buy grocery store rejects. The article "Tampa Bay Farmers Markets Are Lacking Just One Thing: Farmers" may give you more perspective.[25] That is certainly not true for most, but it does happen.

Keep going to the farmers' market, especially if you've never been before. Enjoy the experience, get to know people, and ask questions about where your food comes from. Just realize the vendors at the markets are there to make a profit as well. While you're at it, find other farmers beyond community-supported agriculture (CSA) and farmers' markets to help get a full view of food production. There are many different ways to sell and produce food—and no single "right" answer!

The big questions and food myths:

- *Is local always best?*
- *Food that is grown closer has less environmental impact, right?*

SNOW, FLORIDIAN STRAWBERRIES, AND
NEW ZEALAND APPLES

Local food makes sense, right? Food that's grown closer tastes better, travels fewer miles, and supports the community. My family likes to grow our own veggies, buy beef from a friend, and pick fruit locally and is quite partial to Michigan's red haven peaches and Indiana's cantaloupes.

We also enjoy bananas, but the only time we ever see growing bananas is on spring break in Mexico. Should we only enjoy bananas when we are in Mexico and they're grown on the same resort?

Likewise, my family also enjoys pineapples from Puerto Rico, almonds from California, and strawberries in February from Florida—all thousands of miles away from my kitchen. Is it wrong of me to want fresh fruit for my family when there is snow on the ground? Not necessarily.

Eating local food seems like common sense, until you read *The Locavores Dilemma: In Praise of the 10,000-Mile Diet.* If you're into food, I recommend the book, though it's a very cerebral read. Authors Desrochers and Shimizu summarize "Turning our back on the global food supply chain, and in the process, reducing the quantity of food produced in the most suitable locations will inevitably result in larger amounts of inferior land being put under cultivation."[26]

They point to lower yields and greater environmental damage, as well as the locavores' rejection of technological advancements such as no-till farming. The authors share numerous life cycle assessment studies which have "debunked" locavores' claims about greenhouse gases associated with food miles.

As it turns out, producing food requires a lot more energy than transporting food, particularly if heating or cooling of the products is necessary during transport. For example, shipping freshly picked apples from New Zealand in that country's summer to the United Kingdom during its winter is actually more sustainable because less energy is used in cold storage. Apples grown in the United Kingdom and stored for five to nine months (experiencing normal food loss rates) used 8 to 16 percent more energy in studies cited in *The Locavores Dilemma.*

To quote the authors on the myth of locavorism healing the earth: "A world with modern agriculture will dramatically curtail our impact on the environment. Increased competitive pressures cause farmers to constantly find new and better ways of doing things, including economies of scale, relocating their operations or increasing their purchases from businesses located in more suitable areas—which will spare nature while increasing production."[27]

How much does it cost to heat your house in the dead of winter? The same is true for a greenhouse in New York trying to grow tomatoes. But if those tomatoes are grown in sunlight and shipped in, they are likely to not only taste better, but also require less total energy use.

The same is true for frozen or canned fruits. The USDA's My Plate calls for fruit and vegetables as an essential part of a healthy diet.[28] Canned foods are comparable to cooked and fresh varieties in their nutrient contribution—all provide needed nutrients that make a healthy diet. That does not change whether the produce was grown 25 or 2,500 miles away.

Local is great when it's available. Canned fruit also meets nutrient requirements. So does frozen produce. What matters is you are getting produce on your plate—not whether it was grown in the same zip code or not.

12. Where Fruits Grow, Bugs Go

WHO WANTS BUGS IN THEIR HAIR . . . OR THEIR FRUIT?

Lice. That one word is enough to strike fear in the heart of any parent. In a closed system like a school, lice (which is a blood-sucking bug) spread fairly quickly. The same is true in a closed system like fruit orchards, vineyards, and patches because the ideal host (fruit, trees, bushes) is in a relatively close area.

> **Food Truth**
>
> Chemicals are naturally in food and are needed to protect it.

So I ask you, why is it okay to treat a child's bug-infested head with chemicals and proactively spray their hair with products like peppermint spray, but not protect fruit with similar types of products and chemicals that prevent the spread of disease? It would be ideal to not have to treat either, but we live in a world with bugs.

The big questions and food myths:

- *How can chemicals on my fruit be safe for my family?*
- *Why do farmers apply so many chemicals?*

PLANTS GROW CHEMICALS

Chemicals are bad, right? Nasty manufacturing plants corrupting the environment. The product of giant corporations, designed to poison us? Not quite. Chemicals are a building block of life. All living organisms are usually built from these six chemicals: carbon, hydrogen, nitrogen, oxygen, phosphorous, and sulfur. It is also true that life produces chemicals, such as carbon dioxide.[29]

Plants also make their own pesticides. These have adapted over time and allowed some plants to flourish while others do not. Yes, plants have survival of the fittest and have changed to beat out bugs, fungi, and weeds.

Prior to getting into a discussion of how chemicals are used in food production today, keep the natural elements of chemistry in mind. We are all made up of chemicals—and so is your apple. Did you know an apple contains the chemical amygdalin in its seeds? "Just because a chemical is present, does not mean that it is harmful in the AMOUNT present," says Compound Interest on behalf of Sense About Science.[30]

Although it may seem ideal to grow food without the use of chemicals, it is not realistic. Where fruits grow, bugs flourish. The sugar in fruits acts like an addictive drug for insects that attack fruit in the form of worms, bugs, and larvae. And in the interest of food safety, there is little tolerance by processors, retailers, or consumers for buggy fruit.

Case in point: cherries. Ben LaCross is a second-generation cherry grower in one of the prettiest tips of northern Michigan. His dad started with 40 acres of tart cherries in the 1970s and bought more cherry farms, then starting adding on-farm storage and shipping facilities. They bought controlling interest in Leelanau Fruit Company in 1995 and then other facilities that allowed them to find the equipment to "finish" maraschino cherries and produce fruitcake mixes for large bakeries and cherry mixes used by several ice cream brands.

Ben hopes to pass on the business to his three children. He says he wants to "continue what my father started" and farms because of his family's legacy. He loves the diversity of the things he does, from driving his tractor and working the land to playing in the business world and dabbling in politics. "Raising a family in the best place in the world" is one of Ben's favorite parts of being on a farm.

GROWING PERFECT FRUIT

Ben talks about the process needed to grow the perfect cherry. "There is no room for error, as the processors have a zero tolerance for insects." In a very specialized region (thanks to the Great Lakes) that can easily produce 180 million pounds of cherries per year, there is a lot of draw for bugs.

He points to the question he was asked by a kindergartener when he went to read to their class during National Ag Week. "Why do my dad's cherry trees die every year?" The reality is that there are a lot of threats to fruit trees that easily destroy them.

"It's a lot harder to grow a healthy cherry tree commercially than a tomato plant or any garden. We can't grow a commercially viable cherry orchard without crop protection products." Trees are attacked by root worms and borers, leaves are destroyed by fungus, and the fruit is infested by bugs.

"Fungal diseases are a major problem with fruit crops because they have no immune system to fight off pathogens," Ben says, pointing to leaf spot as an example.

"Trees have to be sprayed for this fungus every seven days since the leaves are growing so quickly. If trees aren't sprayed, they lose their leaves. No leaves, no life."

Just as you would treat ringworm on your skin, fungal diseases on fruit trees are treated with a mix of chemicals and copper products, applied at minimal rates by spraying the trees. The Environmental Protection Agency (EPA) label mandates the last spray is 7 to 14 days before harvest.

Pests start attacking the cherries as soon as the tree puts out fruit. Plum curculio is an insect that uses green fruit to lay its eggs, which hatch into a worm at harvest. Ben pointed to the zero tolerance processors have for this; if one worm is found, all the cherries are wasted. Not only will the processor not accept a load of cherries if a worm is present—the entire orchard will have to be abandoned—a very costly problem.

How do cherry farmers like Ben assure they deliver cherries with no bugs? They spray pesticides. The alternative is no product for maraschino cherries, cherry-baked goods, or cherry ice cream. The pesticides have been extensively researched and are applied at the smallest amount possible—but they are necessary.

"There is a new pest from Japan that has been moving north in Michigan and threatens all of the orchards," Ben said. "This spotted wing drosophila needs a soft fruit like a cherry to host their egg. In four weeks, this bug can go through eight generations. Each female has the ability to lay 300 eggs."

Ben indicates that this one bug threatens the whole cherry business in northern Michigan more so than anything else they have dealt with. He said Michigan State University has been researching it, but has found no chemical that disrupts the life cycle or mating cycle thus far.

Theoretically, three additional pesticide sprays may be needed to control this one bug. Large amounts of money are being poured into research to try to save northern Michigan's cherry business. The goal is to find something to control the bug—natural would be ideal, but a chemical is far more likely in order for cherries to be readily available to you.

The same is true for apples—they're scabby trees if they don't get any help. Apple scab is the biggest threat to the apple business; this is a fungus that defoliates trees and damages the fruit. Damaged fruit attracts more bugs. Bugs make for more blemished apples. And blemished apples contribute to food waste because who wants to buy anything less than a perfect apple?

Jeff Vanderwerff is another Michigander fruit grower who lives and farms with his family close to Lake Michigan. Jeff is a dad to two little girls, is a volunteer fireman, is opinionated about his politics, and is a husband to a scientist working in cancer research. He and his brother raise apples as part of their family partnership with their dad, along with corn and soybeans.

Jeff, one of 7,500 apple producers in the United States, talks about the old way of spraying apples, when a fungicide was sprayed every four days, whether it rained or not. Apples were sprayed every seven days, killing all bugs—good and bad.

INTEGRATED PEST MANAGEMENT, MODELING,
AND MODERATION

"We have since learned that is not the best way to operate, thanks to research at Michigan State University. Integrated pest management is our best tool, though it is very complicated. We now collect temperatures, humidity, dew point, daylight data through fully automated weather systems—while having experts monitor for actual symptoms," Jeff explains. "This is applied to computerized modeling to determine the likelihood of apple scab. We will only treat when the conditions are right for the fungus to grow."

Yes, trees are monitored *that* closely, and farmers apply as little fungicide as possible. In short, growing fruit is complicated. Weather is always the enemy. To put that in perspective, Jeff says it costs him about $15,000 every time it rains. Michigan is a lush, green state—it rains frequently. Imagine gambling against Mother Nature like that. And that doesn't even take all the bugs and wildlife into consideration!

These chemicals are approved by the EPA and USDA; farmers rely on a certified crop advisor and can only use a product at a prescribed rate. If they are mixing approved chemicals, those mixes also have to be at an approved rate. In other words, a farmer cannot mix different chemicals however they want to. It is very specific. There's a lot of self-monitoring that goes on in the farm community, so it becomes pretty clear if one farmer has created some magical recipe.

When I asked Jeff how a grocery shopper would know for sure that our apples are safe from all of these chemicals, he quickly replied, "We are bound by the label. It dictates to us what we can and can't do. There's a time before harvest, we absolutely can't spray, called pre-harvest interval (PHI). Traceability is huge. The risk is not worth going off the label."

Knowing the skepticism that exists about chemical use in food production, I pushed Jeff on the issue. He went on to explain the audit system he has to undergo with Primus Global Audit. He can actually trace an apple back to a block in an orchard and the worker who picked it. Jeff keeps track of pickers within blocks each day and retains records for years, until he is sure every apple is consumed.

Let's say you buy a bag of apples and you get sick after eating one of those apples. The grocery store traces that bag back to the packer, who then traces the apple back to the grower and orchard. The farmer is required to maintain records of what block (small part of the orchard) the apples came from and who picked it. A food safety meeting will be called within hours, and if the problem appears to be a norovirus from the worker, all apples picked by that worker 48 hours beforehand and 48 hours afterwards will be recalled. Likewise, if it is found that some sort of chemical is making people sick, all of the apples from that orchard will be recalled. The farmer will be held liable. As Jeff states again, "The risk is not worth going off the label."

This does not even account for farmer pride in producing healthy food. They want to do the right thing for not only the food buyer, but also the environment. Their family also eats the product. They live on the land. Farmers have a great deal of motivation to grow products the right way.

Consider that kind of traceability with the nearly 170 million bushels of table apples produced across 32 states.[31] The gold standard in food safety for apples is Primus Global Audit, which is required by most packing sheds. In other words, if an apple grower wants to sell table apples, Primus Global Audit is required. Traceability and understanding foodborne risks and standards are a huge part of the audit.

The food safety procedures outlined in Primus Global Audit are 350 pages long and take up a 2-inch-thick three-ring binder. Fifty percent of the binder is policies of how to do things in the orchard. As an example, Jeff mentioned the clippers (like large toenail clippers) that are used to clip stems off of honey crisp apples to prevent stem puncture because of thin skin. "There are 2-1/2 pages about the clippers on their sterilization, use, and the training of employees. The amount of information we are required to know from the book is mind-boggling."

Did you know the only time a bagged apple is touched by a human hand is when it is picked? Water is actually used to move apples at packing. Apples are submerged in a sanitizing minimal bleach solution, which serves to keep the water clean and grab any bacteria off of apples. Once the apples are softly scrubbed, polished, and waxed, they are considered pretty enough to bag.

The wax not only makes the apple look pretty; it hinders the production of ethylene through storage and shipping. Ethylene is known as the aging hormone in plants. It is a naturally occurring small hydrocarbon gas. Apples and pears are examples of fruit that produce ethylene with ripening.[32]

Are chemicals in your fruit? Yes, whether they are organic or conventional. Plants produce chemicals for their own protection. Farmers apply chemicals under heavy scrutiny to further protect the fruit and are careful to follow the label to ensure fruit is not sprayed too close to harvest. Given expectations of having the "perfect" fruit today, it's a necessity.

13. Excuse Me, There's a Cucumber in My Papaya

HEAVENLY HAWAIIAN PAPAYAS

The first time I visited Hawaii and discovered the sweet flesh of papayas, I thought I was in heaven. I had never touched them before in the grocery store since they were kind of foreign looking. You know how it goes: if you don't know what to do with a food, you skip it.

After eating untold quantities of the fleshy orange innards of papaya on the islands, I make it a point to seek

> **Food Truth**
> Genes are the coolest ingredient on your plate.

them out now. Besides being one of my favorite tropical fruits, papaya also make me think about Joni, a friend whose family are papaya farmers.

She's a tiny person with a huge personality. Born and raised in Hawaii, Joni's grandfather and father have both farmed there. Joni said, "I never knew that the story of the Hawaii papaya would have an impact upon the small farmers of the world." She talks openly about how hard it is for her to see farmers not have a voice in the discussion around biotechnology (GMO) at her blog, Hawaii Farmer's Daughter.

Her passion has to do with protecting her family, because their Kamiya papaya farm, along with other farms, was nearly lost to disease in 1990s.

The big questions and food myths:

- *How can it be safe to alter a plant's genetic makeup?*
- *Why would a farmer need genetically modified crops?*

A CUCUMBER GENE SAVES THE DAY

The family farm was saved because of biotechnology. Genetic engineering allowed a family business to be passed on to another generation: Joni's brother, Michael Kamiya.

A devastating ringspot virus hit Hawaii in the 1940s. Papaya growing moved between islands, going from Oahu to Puna, and then the virus was found in back-yards nearby. Aphids spread the virus, which nearly destroyed papaya plants. The result was nearly $17 million lost in papaya business for the islands. Family businesses like the Kamiyas were fighting to survive.[33]

Finding a solution to this became the focus of everyone involved with papayas, to save both family businesses and a major contributor to the Hawaiian economy. A team of researchers tested hundreds of plants to see which were resistant to the virus and chose a cucumber. They identified the gene that was resistant to the ringspot virus from the cucumber and isolated it so they could use it in the papaya.

The solution came from the virus itself—meaning it's like a vaccination we take to avoid chickenpox. Scientists isolated the gene from the cucumber from the virus's protein coat and inserted it into papaya cells. One of the papaya cells added the new gene to its own DNA, which was incorporated into the papaya. It allows the cells' defenses to recognize the virus's gene product as foreign and destroy the virus by chopping it into such small pieces that no infection occurs.[34]

Then came the regulatory agencies, charged with making sure the new virus-resistant papaya was safe for humans and the environment. Animal Plant Health Inspection Services (APHIS) considered the impact on agricultural environments, and the EPA looked at the pesticidal impact of the viral coat protein produced by the transgenic papaya. Finally, the FDA considered the food safety aspect of the transgenic papaya.[35] And the once-endangered papaya plant continued to exist.

In 1997 the U.S. government concluded its regulatory review of the transgenic papaya variety named Rainbow, which includes that gene from a cucumber that makes the papaya plants resistant to the ringspot virus. The genetic improvement allowed production to return to levels similar to before the papaya ringspot virus invaded. Family farms could continue growing papaya for the rest of us to enjoy.

Papaya is unlike most other foods you hear about in the genetically modified organism (GMO) debate; it is not a major commodity. However, in order to successfully grow papaya today in Hawaii today, genetically protecting it from the ringspot virus is essential.

GENES, GENES EVERYWHERE

Genes are in every living being—including you; they're not the bad guy. Remember the pain of picking seeds out of grapes? Thank a gene for your seedless grapes. Enjoy watching your kids bury their face in watermelon with no worry of choking on seeds? Thank a gene for your seedless watermelon.

Researcher Kevin Folta, whose lab at the University of Florida uses genomics techniques to identify genes driving important crop traits, explains how breeding seedless watermelons is a genetic cross. There is an actual transfer of pollen from one type of watermelon to another. "Polyploids are defined as organisms that contain many more than the normal number of chromosomes. In plants, it is common to find instances where the chromosomes have doubled, meaning two sets from the female and two sets from the male, four sets all together. The extra genetic material is not a problem and in many cases, it helps create larger fruits with better quality.

"Now imagine if you cross a polyploid watermelon (two sets of chromosomes from the female) with a diploid (one set from the male). The resulting offspring will be triploid (one too many chromosome sets). This odd set of chromosomes is tough for a plant cell to understand, and so the cells don't develop, and the seeds are unviable."[36] Does that make seedless watermelon bad for you?

Another great example of genes at work is the Arctic apple, which was developed in British Columbia, Canada. This apple doesn't brown as fast because they have slowed down the gene that causes browning of the apple. I don't know about you, but no matter how many times I try to talk myself into eating those leftover brown apple slices—they still kind of gross me out. Arctic apples have suppressed polyphenol oxidase (PPO) production. PPO is the naturally occurring enzyme that makes apples brown, as well as lettuce and mushrooms. Four little genes stop that from happening through gene editing.[37] Yes, genes are on your plate—and they are amazing!

The World Health Organization defines GMOs as "organisms (i.e., plants, animals or microorganisms) in which the genetic material (DNA) has been altered in a way that does not occur naturally by mating and/or natural recombination."

The technology is often called "modern biotechnology" or "gene technology," sometimes also "recombinant DNA technology" or "genetic engineering." It allows selected individual genes to be transferred from one organism into another and also between nonrelated species. Foods produced from or using GM organisms are often referred to as GM foods."[38]

Chromosomes and DNA do belong in your food—and genes can be the coolest ingredient on your plate, if you take a couple of minutes to understand them instead of fear them. Dr. Jason Lusk from Oklahoma State University conducted a study showing 80 percent of Americans believe DNA in their food should be labeled.[39] Why? Everything that came from a live plant or animal contains chromosomes, genes, and DNA. Genes can do amazing things, from protecting a plant for long-term survival, to offering more nutrition in a piece of fruit, making it more convenient for those of us who enjoy fruit.

14. Cutting Boards and Cross-Contamination

WHEN LIFE GIVES YOU LEMONS . . .

Lemon slices give your drink a boost of flavor, but they may also offer a whole host of other things. In fact, a 2007 study found that nearly 70 percent of restaurant lemon wedges are covered in up to 25 different types of germs and other organic material. Among them: fecal matter, *E. coli*, and contamination from raw meat. And it wasn't just the lemon rinds—the pulp on 29 percent of the dirty lemons was crawling in bacteria, too.[40]

> **Food Truth**
>
> Food safety starts on the farm and ends in your kitchen.

Lemons could be contaminated for a number of reasons. While you might be diligent enough to scrub your lemons at home, there's no guarantee that the wait staff is washing every single one to perfection or that they have washed their hands after their bathroom break. Couple that with a restaurant potentially using the same knives for cutting raw meat and produce, and contamination can quickly spread.

Lemons and other citrus (we're looking at you, limes) are especially susceptible because they are covered in pores, giving bacteria extra surface area to dig into. The same study concluded that microorganisms can survive on the flesh and rind of a sliced lemon—meaning you should be aware that lemon slices added to your drink "may include potentially pathogenic microbes."

Don't get me wrong; lemons and limes and all other types of citrus are lovely. I enjoy them as a real way to freshen up my drinks. But only if I buy them and cut them. After all, you don't know whose hands—and bacteria—have been in your food.

The big questions and food myths:

- *Why are people getting sick from fruit?*
- *How can I protect my family with food safety?*

SKIP THE ANTIBACTERIAL SOAPS AND HAND SANITIZERS

Bacteria are bad, right? Gross little creatures that make us sick? Not quite; there are good and bad bacteria. You need some to maintain a healthy digestive system, yet others can kill you.

Bacteria are microscopic living organisms, usually one celled, found everywhere. And yes, your gut houses a whole bunch of them![41] They even are even under your fingernails and all over your skin; you're actually the host to about a trillion bacteria. Bacteria can make you sick or be beneficial, such as those in your gut.

Interestingly enough, antibacterial soaps don't necessarily solve the handwashing problem. The FDA announced in 2014 that manufacturers have to show over-the-counter antibacterial soap is both safe and more effective than conventional hand washing.

According to Colleen Rogers, PhD, a lead microbiologist at the FDA, there is no evidence these products are more effective at preventing illness than washing with plain soap and water. Antibacterial soap products contain chemical ingredients, such as tricolosan and triclocarban, which may carry unnecessary risks. Canada banned soaps with triclosan.

"New data suggests that risks associated with the long-term daily use of antibacterial soaps may outweigh the benefits," Rogers says. "There are indications that certain ingredients in these soaps may contribute to bacterial resistance to antibiotics, and may have unanticipated hormonal effects that are of concern to the FDA."[42]

GO BACK TO THE BASICS; WASH YOUR HANDS

Given the amount of antibacterial use among the mom crowd, this could cause a bit of hysteria. No need. There's a simple answer. Wash your hands with soap for 15 to 20 seconds. It's simple.

"Clean hands save lives" is the Centers for Disease Control's (CDC's) mantra. They indicate washing hands with soap and warm water is the best way to reduce the number of microbes in most situations. If soap and water are not available, use an alcohol-based sanitizer that contains at least 60 percent alcohol. Although alcohol-based hand sanitizers quickly reduce the number of microbes in some situations, they do *not* eliminate all types of germs. They also don't remove chemicals from hands.

Turns out the same is true for your fruit, but skip the soap—and the alcohol, lest we be dipping our fruit in vodka. The FDA does *not* recommend washing produce with soap, detergent, bleach, or commercial washes. Rather:

- Handle produce with care to minimize bruising
- Wash in cold water
- Dry off any excess water
- Keep produce that is supposed to be kept cool in the refrigerator (set at 40 degrees Fahrenheit or below)
- Dispose of any fruits or vegetables that look like they are going bad

Washing your fruit and handling it properly goes a long way toward food safety. Don't assume fruit are laden with chemicals; the farm stories shared earlier in this chapter illustrate there are rigorous withholding times for many pesticide and fungicide applications. In other words, they can't be sprayed right before harvest, and the fruit is certainly not "drenched" in chemicals, as some claim.

What's that waxy feel on your apple? Food-grade wax put on at the packing house to help preserve the apple. What's the white stuff on your grapes? A harmless coating that the grape plant naturally produces to keep moisture in the grapes. Wash and wipe; these substances will go away.

FERMENTED OR ROTTEN FRUIT?

Bacteria can also help ferment food, which has positive application, like wine or hard cider. Fermentation of grapes caused by bacteria is actually pretty cool. What makes the difference between that molding mush formerly known as a grape in the back of your refrigerator and the lovely pinot in your wine cabinet? Selective science in a controlled environment.

There is also the bad side to bacteria, usually in a less controlled environment, such as when your fruit decomposes into brown mush in the back of your refrigerator.

The bacteria causing fruit and vegetable spoilage actually won't harm humans, though they can make the produce mushy, which is more attractive to human pathogens such as Salmonella.

E. coli and Listeria are another example of bacteria that cause human illness. These are the bacteria that can make you sick. You can see a list of foodborne illness investigations at http://www.cdc.gov/foodsafety/outbreaks/multistate-outbreaks /outbreaks-list.html.

No system is perfect, including agriculture. However, it's good to know there are benchmarks and audits protecting your fruit. I asked Ryan Van Groningen out in California about keeping melons safe from bugs and bacteria.

"Since a majority of our acreage is grown conventionally or traditionally, we rely on herbicides [weed control], insecticides, fungicides, etc., to keep our plants safe from anything that might affect their growing negatively. We *only* use chemicals that have been approved by the FDA, USDA, and EPA. And we apply to a certain crop and only apply them at rates that have been tested to cause no harm to the consumer."

At some point, a consumer has to balance if they are more comfortable with pesticide use in food production or the potential for bacteria. I always go with what science supports, which means I'm okay with pesticides used responsibly, but not bacteria.

WHAT'S THE STANDARD IN IMPORTED FRUIT PRODUCTION?

In the United States, more protocols are in place today than there ever have been. I'm much more comfortable with the food production standards in developed countries like the United States, Australia, and Canada than I am with what is done in developing countries.

According to the USDA, the United States consumed 635 billion pounds of food in 2013. That's one ton (2,000 pounds) per person. Nearly 20 percent of the food was imported—and that number is growing. I believe part of the food safety question needs to be about the standards for imported food. Is it grown the same way, and are there audits in place? Are the same regulations followed in other countries? From my experience, not always.

Whether it's in the fruit aisle or with meats served at a restaurant, we need to consider food safety. If we continue to put so much pressure on farmers to produce more with less while increasing regulations, we will be importing significantly more food.

As I select fruit, I know that the last step in the safety of my food lies in my hands in my kitchen. Washing my fruit properly, not exposing it to knives or cutting surfaces used with meats, and remembering to wash my hands before handling my fruit greatly reduce my family's exposure.

15. Organic Produce Requires Pesticides?

THE REAL DIRT IN THE
DIRTY DOZEN

Are you aware of the Dirty Dozen list? It's a "consumer guide" that I call the celebrity list of fruits and vegetables that you should *never* buy unless they're organic. Turns out the real dirt is the group behind the Dirty Dozen, known as the Environmental Working Group (EWG).

According to ActivistFacts.com, 79 percent of members of the Society of Toxicology rating EWG say that the

> **Food Truth**
>
> Organic farming is about production methods, not nutritional value.

group overstates the health risk of chemicals. In the Dirty Dozen list, the EWG publicizes what they call "dirty" pesticide residues on fruits and vegetables. The problem is that the EWG never mentions that the "dirty" pesticide levels are actually safe because they're well below the "tolerance" levels set by the EPA.[43]

The big questions and food myths:

- *Isn't organic fruit safer?*
- *Aren't chemicals in fruit bad?*
- *Should I feel guilty if I don't buy organic?*

FEAR THE FORMALDEHYDE!

Did you know that a pear contains 40 to 60 mg/kg of formaldehyde?[44] Sounds awful, doesn't it? Some could read that and derive that pears are washed in formaldehyde. A social media meme would be created, national headlines would be made, and people would fear the pear.

Pears aren't washed in formaldehyde, but they do produce the chemical on their own. So do you! All life forms naturally produce formaldehyde in cell metabolism.[45] It's not bad—it's just life!

So what if pear baby food was labeled as containing formaldehyde, or by its chemical formula CH_2O (it's made up of hydrogen, oxygen, and carbon)? As a mom trying to make the right food choice for my family, I certainly would never have bought that baby food.

Yet formaldehyde is an organic substance. It is a chemical that is produced by life. It is necessary for life.

BT AS AN ORGANIC PESTICIDE, BUT CONDEMNED AS A GMO

Did you know a naturally occurring bacterium is a commonly used insecticide? First isolated in Japan in 1901 and then by a German scientist again in 1915, *Bacillus thuringiensis (Bt)* has a crystal that makes the bacteria an insecticide.[46]

Insecticidal proteins produced by *Bt* are used as a spray in organic farming. Genes from the exact same protein have been incorporated into several major crops through genetic engineering. One is a spray applied to crops for organic production; the other is incorporated into the plant so sprays will not have to be applied. Is one right and the other wrong?

The *Bt* bacteria have provided a uniquely specific, safe, and effective tool for the control of a wide variety of insect pests. *Bt* has been used in spray formulations for over 40 years, where it is considered remarkably safe, in large part because specific formulations harm only a narrow range of insect species. Today, *Bt* insecticidal protein genes have been incorporated into several major crops, providing a model for agricultural genetic engineering.[47]

As an example, *Bt* is labeled for use in apples to prevent leaf rollers (a type of insect) in organic production. According to Michigan apple grower Jeff mentioned in Chapter 12, one pound of *Bt* insecticide can be used for organic apple production, compared with two ounces of synthetic insecticide used in a regular apple orchard. That's a rate that is eight times higher for the organic product.

Further, *Bt* is not approved for organic corn growers. Products engineered with the exact same insecticidal protein are condemned by the organic community for that different commodity. That also makes me question the claims—if it can be used at a heavy rate as an insecticide in apples, why is it wrong when it's in a corn seed?

Don't get me wrong; I support organic farmers and believe they have a right to choose the best market for their family. Organic foods have gained popularity; there is a clear perception that organic foods are safer and more nutritious. Again, I question the science and ask how much is marketing.

WHAT DOES ORGANIC MEAN?

Organic farming is a food production process. It is defined by the USDA, and producers who want to use the USDA organic label on their food must be certified. They have to comply with federal regulations, just as conventional producers do. Both types of farmers must follow rules for safe production practices. Both care for the soil. Both organic and conventional foods are inspected. Both control pests. Both types of production are regulated and monitored for safety when it comes to levels of chemicals, pesticides and antibiotics.

The organic crop production standards require that:

- Land must have had no prohibited substances applied to it for at least three years before the harvest of an organic crop.
- Soil fertility and crop nutrients will be managed through tillage and cultivation practices, crop rotations, and cover crops, supplemented with animal and crop waste materials and allowed synthetic materials.
- Crop pests, weeds, and diseases will be controlled primarily through management practices, including physical, mechanical, and biological controls. When these practices are not sufficient, a biological, botanical, or synthetic substance approved for use on the National List may be used.[48]

Qualifying to produce organic produce is a long waiting period. It's interesting to note that certain pesticides are approved, as long as they are on the National List. As a plant pathologist and horticulturist with Colorado State University outlined about growing produce, "If we think organic gardening means vegetables free of any chemical pesticides, we don't have the story quite right. Organic gardeners can use certain pesticides—chemicals that are derived from botanical and mineral-bearing sources. These chemicals may be highly toxic . . ." Just like with other production methods, there is a large difference in organic farms; there are some who use nothing and others who will use all the tools available to them.

Some of the botanical and mineral-based pesticides allowed in organic production include nicotine sulfate, sulfur, sabadilla, neem, and lime sulfur, which have varying levels of toxicity, the same as chemicals used in conventional farming. A complete list of synthetic substances allowed in the National Organic Program can be found at the "Electronic Code of Federal Regulations" at the U.S. Government Publishing Office.[49]

ISN'T ORGANIC PRODUCE MORE NUTRITIOUS?

Do you assume foods not labeled organic are less nutritious and may even contain harmful chemicals, pesticides, and antibiotics? Research shows otherwise.

"There is very little evidence showing significant differences in nutritional value of organic and conventional foods," according to Ruth MacDonald, professor and chair of the Department of Food Science and Human Nutrition at Iowa State University.[50]

She points out, "Controlled research studies of organic and conventional goods using sensory analysis have been conducted with no differences in perception of taste found. It's also important to note there are many other factors that influence the quality and taste of foods, such as freshness, storage conditions, variety of the crop or product, and, of course, personal preference. Research studies show organic foods do not provide special nutritional or safety benefits and conventional foods are nutritious and healthful."

I was speaking at a food conference, where dietitians questioned the sustainability of organic compared with conventional farming. They were surprised to learn organic produce can have pesticides used. These healthcare professionals also seemed shocked to learn the difference in productivity and potential implications of organic's lower yield requiring more land. Sustainability in food production is far more complex than only looking at a single factor, such as pesticides.

At the end of the day, your fruit selection comes down to choice. All fruits have chemicals in them, are raised with some sort of pest protection, and are nutritious. You choose what is right for your family; that's a decision that should not be driven by guilt. The good news is that we have choice; you can likely find food to fit whatever philosophy you want.

There is no singular right way to raise produce. There is no singular right way to purchase produce. The good news? There's a solid system in place to protect you whether you buy organic or conventional fruit.

16. Water and Family: The Lifeblood of Growing Food

SOLAR-POWERED CRANBERRIES

Three generations working side by side to bring in harvest. Identical twin daughters. Long days of staring at little red berries, followed by short nights. Energy, patience, stamina, and passion are needed to bring in this tangy holiday tradition.

> **Food Truth**
>
> Sustainability is complex and essential to family businesses.

Fall harvest in Massachusetts is a beautiful combination of crimson color on this cranberry farm and colorful foliage, bringing joy to the long days, according to Dawn Gates-Allen, who farms with her family.

And it's a life Dawn wouldn't trade for anything. She's a working mom, but her office involves tall boots and a lot of water. And solar-powered sensors talk to her laptop—wherever it might be. Those sensors make sure the cranberries don't get beyond 105 degrees in their bogs and have enough moisture.

The next time you drink cranberry juice, enjoy a handful of Craisins, or cook with cranberries, consider this: your cranberries have to float to be harvested. And there's a whole lot of focus on the environment to get them to that point.

Agriculture that doesn't prioritize sustainability is an unrealistic myth. To infer farmers and ranchers are not invested in sustainability reflects a lack of firsthand familiarity with today's food production practices.

The big questions and food myths:

- *Is growing produce really sustainable?*
- *Wouldn't it be better for the environment if we all had a garden?*

WATER IS THE LIFEBLOOD OF A SUSTAINABLE FAMILY BUSINESS

Dawn, her husband, and twin daughters are the only labor you'll find on their 27 acres of cranberry bogs most of the year. Dawn's parents and two brothers pool their labor during harvest of their mutual bogs. The girls are the fifth-generation cranberry growers.

Size doesn't define the farm. Family does.

Protecting the environment is a top priority for cranberry farmers. Dawn and her husband have invested hundreds of thousands of dollars in conservation upgrades, including pop-up sprinklers, automated irrigation, and new water control flumes. Solar energy gives constant battery power to the automated irrigation receivers, saving 15 percent in fuel annually.

Water is literally the lifeblood and is recycled throughout the bog system. Water provides frost protection in spring and fall, protects root zones during the harshest winter months, and is essential to harvest.

"It's a privilege to be a farmer and take care of our land." Dawn shares. That care is such a concern that they use food-grade oils in the harvesting equipment because if something does happen, they have equipment to contain and clean up the spill.

Moving to the opposite side of the country, there are few places that have been challenged by environmentalists like California. Van Groningen and Sons, fourth-generation farmers, started farming there in 1922 with a dairy operation; moved to row crops; and today are known for melons, sweet corn, gourds, pumpkins, and almonds.

"We do not recycle water, but we do preserve water. All of our fields and ranches use drip irrigation, which considerably lowers the amount of water a crop uses," said Ryan Van Groningen.

"Growers definitely must make decisions on what they will grow and how many acres, depending on water availability. At times, growers will need to fallow prime farmland because they do not have enough water to provide for all of the acreage, if planted."

Water is a critical factor in the business of growing fruit and vegetables, many of which come from the West Coast. Van Groningen & Sons farms around 5,000 acres in Manteca, California, where, as mentioned, they grow melons, sweet corn, pumpkins, and nuts. It sounds like a huge business, but seven family member owners maintain an active daily role, along with 50 full-time employees.

"Big ag" often comes up as a food concern, so I asked Ryan if they still consider themselves a family farm. He said, adamantly, "Yes, we are definitely a family farm. We are owned and operated by the Van Groningen family and do not have any outside investors."

Water is the lifeblood of both of these family farms, large and small, West Coast and East Coast. Sustainability is a driving business concern to farmers and ranchers—and since their families are involved with the land and water on a daily basis, it's personal. Protecting their business for future generations is also a part of the sustainability model.

FAMILY DEFINES THE FARM

Family is at the heart and soul of farming—whether it's cranberry bogs, cantaloupe fields, or cows. I spent some time talking with friend Jolene Brown about sustainable family businesses, and she summed it up perfectly from 30 years of speaking to and working with farm families: "Family business includes a 'genetic group' of individuals who want to honor the family by doing the business right. They believe in the purpose of what they do and they do it with great stewardship and passion."

It's frustrating for farmers to hear "big ag" or "industrial farming" or similar terms. It's the same families growing and raising food, with the same values. Jolene pointed out, "Ninety-seven percent of all farms and ranches are family businesses today. Farms and ranches are structured into entities like corporations to do two things: incrementally transition the business to continue the legacy and to take responsibility for liability. Our big corporate farm is two people: Keith and Jolene."

I asked her why she farmed. "First, farming reinforces our family value system. Secondly, there is national security in agriculture. I don't want to be dependent on another country for our food supply. Finally, I love my farmer. This is his heart, it his mind, it is his labor, it is his joy."

Sustainability is "not just renewal, it's making what you have better for the next generation. Sustainability is understanding the limitations and opportunities of a resource, such as knowing the role of micronutrients to make your land better and looking for ways to reduce soil erosion, like a buffer strip," she explained.

As you grab a bag of fruit or nuts during your next produce department visit, my hope is that you will consider farm families like these that are thinking about sustainability on a daily basis. They may define it differently than a label on your food, but sustainability remains a priority.

Table 3   Fruit Food Truths

Food Myth	Food Truth
Buying food locally helps the environment.	**Food Truth 8: Local is not always better for the environment.** The energy required to raise food outside of a native environment sometimes trumps food miles when it comes to environmental costs.
Chemicals on fruit are poisoning your family.	**Food Truth 9: Chemicals are naturally in food and are needed to protect it.** Where fruit grows, pests thrive. Apples without worms and cherries without bugs require chemicals. And chemicals aren't all bad—they're naturally in food.
Messing with the genetics in food is wrong.	**Food Truth 10: Genes are the coolest ingredient on your plate.** Seedless grapes, papayas, and seedless watermelon are all products of understanding—and improving—genetics.
Today's farming methods make my fruit unsafe.	**Food Truth 11: Food safety starts on the farm and ends in your kitchen.** Proper washing of fruit in water and keeping bacteria off your cutting surfaces goes a long way in protecting your family—as does the intense traceability of fruit.
Organic fruit is the only right choice for my family.	**Food Truth 5: Organic farming is about production methods, not nutritional value.** Getting your fruit is more important than the way it was produced, and many of us lack enough servings of fruit each day.
Growing produce is destroying the environment.	**Food Truth 12: Sustainability is complex and essential to family businesses.** Environmental audits, technology, and family business survival skills all make up a model that is sustainable for generations.

Part IV: Vegetables

What's growing in your vegetable drawer? Thirty-five billion genes in carrots and seemingly nearly as many chemicals used. "Larry the Cucumber" didn't tell me he could be grown in water or that GPS was part of his life. What's happening with vegetable production, where it's coming from, and what any parent needs to know about vegetable power.

"The great enemy of truth is very often not the lie—deliberate, contrived and dishonest—but the myth—persistent, persuasive, and unrealistic. Too often we hold fast to the clichés of our forebears. We subject all facts to a prefabricated set of interpretations. We enjoy the comfort of opinion without the discomfort of thought."

—JFK

17. Does Eating Healthy Cost More?

THE RISK OF GROWING FOOD

Have you ever gardened? If so, you likely recognize how finicky vegetables can be. They want a certain amount of warmth, enough rain—but not too much—and are overly attractive to bugs. Given the hours I have spent in a garden, I'm always amazed by the beautiful produce we find in the store—particularly given the financial risk involved.

> **Food Truth**
>
> Food costs are a shared concern.

Consider this; you decide to invest $100,000 in stocks. Those stocks are controlled by Mother Nature and if it rains at the right time in the right amount. Too much or too little, and the price changes 20 percent. Further, the stocks require around $500,000 in equipment, a cost that can be spread across 10 years. But diesel fluctuates 35 percent for the year, raising your costs. And then the government reduces your water supply by 15 percent mid-season and institutes a new regulation, adding 120 hours of paperwork requirements, which raises both your water and labor costs.

Doesn't sound like a winning proposition for your $100,000 investment, does it? Yet, it is a typical scenario on a farm and ranch—without even considering the costs of planting or raising a crop (which are called input costs). And instead of $100,000 at risk, a family farm risks millions of dollars. Although farming and ranching is a way of life, it is also a business.

Let's look at a vegetable grower example. Hypothetically, a tomato harvester is roughly $500,000. Land costs at least $8,000 an acre to buy. Labor, seeds, and input may cost $100 an acre. If you farm 100 acres of tomatoes, that's more than $1 million risked—by one family, against Mother Nature and a volatile market with a highly perishable product. It can be a terrifying business proposition, one in which farmers are the price takers, not the price makers. That is the daily reality of farmers.

In order to keep that food affordable, efficiency and reduced costs at the farm gate are key. If you wonder why farms are getting larger, it is because the business of farming requires that costs be spread over more acres.

The big questions and food myths:

- *Are farmers getting rich?*
- *Why is fresh food so expensive?*
- *How can I reduce my produce bill?*

CONSERVING COSTS, CHEMICALS, AND TIME

I asked Ryan Van Groningen, who grows sweet corn, melons, pumpkins, and almonds in California, "What do you do to keep the costs of food production and/ or costs of produce in the grocery store as low as possible?"

> Not only is cutting costs beneficial for a business to be more profitable, but typically a very sustainable action on a grower's part as well. We never want to be wasteful, we strive to be conservative. For example, we *never* want to apply extra chemicals to any crop. We only apply the rates and amounts we decide are needed to keep our crop safe and to perform to the best of its abilities. We also are very mindful how a field can have different issues happening in only certain areas of the field so we don't 'prescribe a medicine' for the entire field, only where we see the symptoms, etc.
>
> We are always trying to become more efficient as well. What that means for our operation is we continue to try and find avenues to become more mechanized. That is definitely a possible way to be more efficient and save costs over the long term but also alleviates our ever-growing issue with finding enough labor.
>
> Lastly, another way to keep costs down at the grocery store that a grower can help with is by making sure they are good growers and getting the highest yields possible. For example, you can typically spend $5,000 per acre in growing costs for a melon. If you get 25 to 35 tons per acre, it will definitely change what your cost per pound was to produce.

WHAT ABOUT IMPORTED PRODUCE?

According to the USDA Economic Research Service, the dollar depreciated 24 percent from 2002 to 2011 in price-adjusted terms. However, the cost of imported foods inflated at a faster pace—from 58 cents in 2002 to 95 cents per pound in 2013. Imported foods costs rose 64 percent in 11 years. Consider what that means to your grocery cart.

The import share for tropical products such as bananas, mangos, coffee, cocoa, tea, spices, olive oil, and tropical oils are at or near 100 percent because domestic production is close to zero. Our demand for fresh fruits and vegetables year round, fish, coffee, and meat to meet certain restaurant requirements, along with a greater variety of wines, beers, and grain products, means more food is being imported. Other examples of highly import-dependent products include cashew nuts, pecans, apple juice, table grapes, melons, and fresh tomatoes.[51]

WHY DOES ORGANIC PRODUCE COST MORE?

The Rousseau family has roots in the Salt River Valley dating back to 1878, and Rousseau Farming Company was established in 1979. They believe Arizona, specifically Maricopa County, has a great climate and favorable soil conditions for winter vegetables.

Will Rousseau says the farm grows several thousand acres of both organic and conventional crops.

"Organic is more expensive to harvest because the yields can be lower, and the uniform consistency of a crop can be less in organic. In a conventional field we might be able to harvest a field by going through once or twice and harvest everything, whereas in an organic field we might have to go into the field multiple times to capture the harvestable product.

"Also, an organic product can't be cooled or packed on the same machines after conventional without a complete cleaning. It adds to the packing and cooling costs of a facility when you are running both conventional and organic," he said.

Knowing how it can seem so expensive to eat healthy, I asked what Rousseau Farming Company does to keep the costs of food production low to keep costs of produce in the grocery store as low as possible.

Will explained, "We are constantly re-evaluating our farming practices to increase yields. More product we can harvest off of a piece of land drives down our costs and in turn means cheaper food for consumers. As regulations keep changing, it makes it more and more difficult to produce cheap food. Labor costs, transportation costs, government regulations, healthcare costs, machinery, and land prices are all functions of our costs that we have to recoup back in order to stay in business. The resources and tools we use to farm continue to drive up our costs.

"New varieties are being developed by seed companies and universities to help us stay ahead of diseases and produce high-yielding crops. Each season we conduct extensive trialing on new seed varieties in coordination with our seed companies to confirm we are using the newest and best varieties for our commodities."

HOW CAN I REDUCE MY PRODUCE BILL?

The *Dietary Guidelines* recommend filling half your plate with vegetables and fruit. How can you do that and still keep your food costs within reason? "Keep frozen, canned and dried fruit and vegetables on hand, especially when fresh produce isn't in season. Buy canned fruit that's packed in juice for less added sugars and calories, and choose low-sodium canned vegetables," recommends the Academy of Nutrition and Dietetics.

Frozen foods are a quick and easy way to add an affordable nutritional boost to your meals. *Today's Dietitian* reports people who utilize frozen vegetables are more likely to meet their requirement. Further, frozen and canned vegetable nutrients are comparable to fresh.[52]

If you're like the average American family, you throw away around $1,500 of food each year. Considering how you can get nutrition from produce and not have it rot in your refrigerator is a very real way to reduce your food costs.

18. Vegetables Make Chemicals?

CANCER IS PERSONAL, NOT A DR. OZ SHOW

I will likely never forget the day Mark and I were engaged. But not for the reasons you might guess. Four hours after Mark popped the question and placed a beautiful princess-cut diamond on my finger, his doctor called. "We have concerns about a mass in Mark's right shoulder after reviewing his MRI," the doctor quietly said.

> **Food Truth**
>
> Chemicals are naturally in food and are needed to protect it.

It was the Friday before Christmas, and we had been filled with celebratory joy, but the lights immediately became a lot dimmer. What was supposed to be a rotator cuff tear turned into the toughest news faced by a widower who had lost his first wife to breast cancer. It was a time of heartbreak for us.

Three days later, we were sitting in the office of the best orthopedic oncologist we could find. After a lot of talking, the doctor uttered the word "lymphoma." The doctor talked about the tests; a computed tomography (CT) scan and blood work. He talked about the likely prognosis. When I asked how a vibrant, healthy man ended up with non-Hodgkin's diffuse B-cell lymphoma, the oncologist said there were a lot of different possible reasons: "Environment, injury, pesticide exposure, or genetics could be why one cell became cancerous and then rapidly divides—but no one really knows for certain."

Not having an answer did not give either of us comfort, in spite of the fact that they told us it was curable. However, the doctor's words "No one really knows for certain" were a return to reason with his encouragement to focus on the cure. A known leader in his field was clear that there was no one reason for a normal cells turning into lymphoma.

Wouldn't our world be simpler if more people—especially those with far less expertise than a doctor who manages a bone marrow transplant team—would openly admit there is no single reason for terrible illnesses like cancer? Wouldn't the discussion become more reasonable if people didn't get so hung up on one-sided information? Wouldn't we have a society less likely to turn to sensationalism if opinions weren't held up as fact?

For example, *The Doctor Oz Show* is one of the top five talk shows in the United States, hosted by Dr. Mehmet Oz. "Cancer," he told the *New Yorker*, "is our Angelina Jolie. We could sell that show every day." I don't know which is sadder—that people are "buying" such sensationalism, a doctor considers a disease in terms of marketability, or cancer is being used for selling. It disgusts me.

Cancer sucks. However, no matter how awful a disease is, it is unreasonable to blame every chemical as the reason for it.

Award-winning Berkeley biologist Bruce Ames insisted in a 1995 interview with *Vegetarian Times* magazine that "99.99 percent of the pesticides we eat are naturally present in plants to ward off insects and other predators . . . reducing our exposure to the 0.01 percent of ingested pesticides that are synthetic is not likely to reduce cancer rates."

Like everyone, I hope and pray for an answer for cancer but refuse to turn away from science in spite of cancer becoming very personal.

The big questions and food myths:

- *Are pesticides used in growing my food?*
- *How can chemicals be okay for my family?*
- *What is done to vegetables in the field?*

EVERYTHING IS POISON

Did you know both potatoes and zucchini contain natural chemicals that are toxic to humans? A dried shiitake mushroom contains a huge amount of naturally occurring formaldehyde.[53]

Just because a chemical is present does not mean it is harmful. The amount of the chemical is what makes a chemical toxic! Everything in food truly is science.

"Chemical toxicity is a sliding scale, not black and white—and whether a chemical is naturally occurring or man-made tells us nothing about its toxicity," says Sense About Science, a UK-based charitable trust whose mission is "to equip people to make sense of science and evidence."

A first-hand example of this in food production is seen with the Arizona family farm, Rousseau Farming, which grows both conventional and organic vegetables, including carrots, broccoli, cabbage, dry onions, watermelons, celery, sweet corn, parsley, kale, cilantro, beets, leeks, cauliflower, and chards. They farm around 9,000 acres with 6,500 acres in vegetable crops. They also grow silage corn, wheat, oats, and alfalfa just north of Phoenix.

Will Rousseau's farm is unique, as they grow large quantities of both organic and conventional produce. What are the big differences between growing organic and conventional produce? Is one better than the other?

"The most significant difference is the types of fertilizers and pesticides we are allowed to use. No synthetic fertilizers or pesticides can be used in the production of organic products. However, that does not mean we do not use pesticides or fertilizers in organics; the source is just different. We use fertilizers sourced from animal products and pesticides that are derived from plants, animals, etc.

"Crops, including vegetables, still need a supply of nitrogen, phosphorus, and potassium to grow—therefore the fertilizers are important to their growth and crop yield. Usually the animal-derived products for fertilizer break down in the soil faster and therefore have to be applied closer to planting than a synthetic pre-plant fertilizer would to be sure the roots receive the nutrients. Organic farming does not produce the same yields as a conventionally grown product, so it would be difficult to continue to feed a growing population with the current organic methods," said Will Rousseau.

"There is not one way that is better than the other, comparing organic and conventional. They are different in how you can treat diseases or insect pressure.

"Organic is more expensive to grow because there is a limited amount of available options for inputs to use and when there are crop problems (insects, diseases) that are sometimes more difficult to solve on organic crops with organic solutions."

Bugs love vegetables just as much as they love fruit.

WOULD YOU LIKE SOME MILDEW WITH YOUR GREEN BEANS?

Jennifer Schmidt is a registered dietitian who farms with her husband in the opposite corner of the country from Rousseaus in Maryland. She explains mildew is a huge challenge with the rain and humidity of Maryland summers. Copper and sulfur are used as mildew preventatives across all their fruits and vegetables. In addition to green beans for the fresh market, they grow tomatoes, wine grapes, barley, wheat corn, and soybeans.

"We spray a fungicide like copper sulfate every couple of weeks on the tomatoes and grapes to protect the foliage. Plants with leaves destroyed by fungus are a problem. Nothing ripens if a plant doesn't photosynthesize," says Jennifer. Think back to third-grade science: a plant without leaves cannot photosynthesize.

Consider a terrarium, where plants are in a closed system (like a glass dome). They photosynthesize (convert light energy into chemical energy), releasing water and oxygen. If the system is not right, the plant grows a mold or fungus, which kills it. The same is true for vegetable and fruit plants in fields.

The Schmidts use very little weed control (herbicides) with green beans because they are typically planted immediately after barley or wheat. Jennifer says, "Both of these grains have a dense stubble left after harvest, plus combining (harvesting) the grain heads leaves a lot of chaff (fine grounds from harvesting), which blocks weed growth. Green beans only take a couple of months from planting until harvesting, so they are a fairly quick crop to grow."

Both the Virginia distributor and Pennsylvania tomato cannery that contracts the Schmidts to grow green beans and tomatoes require their water to be tested for bacteria yearly, due to the Food Safety Modernization Act (FSMA). Another food safety measure is that the beans can't be planted within a certain number of feet of cattle due to raw manure. The Schmidt family raises around 1 million bushels of green beans on 100 acres.

TOMATOES ARE A NEEDY CROP

How do you think it would work to sell 7.2 million pounds of tomatoes at farmers' markets? Not well, according to the farmer who grows them, which is why the Schmidts contract with a processor in Pennsylvania. This not only gives them a set market, but also provides planting, harvesting, and trucking for tomatoes. "Otherwise we couldn't cash flow growing vegetables," reports Jennifer.

She describes tomatoes as "a needy crop." They started to grow them to diversify their farm after their neighbor had done so. "It was very different and a steep learning curve. Tomatoes need a regular preventative program like copper sulfate and other crop protection because of rain and humidity." Delivering tomatoes without rot is top priority, as tolerance is less than 2 percent on a semi load or the entire load will be rejected. This is judged by appearance or smell at the cannery.

Consequently, there is a 7- to 10-day spray schedule for most of the season with fungicides to prevent blight, as well as a regular insecticide schedule. "There is no drum of chemicals in the barn that is rolled out and sprayed willy-nilly. It is an exact science, carefully monitored," Jennifer explains.

Prior to harvest in late August, she says, "we use a ripening agent because a mechanical harvester harvests everything. A growth stimulator is sprayed on 10 days ahead of time to help them photosynthesize. This allows for more uniformity because it is a growth regulator."

19. Freshness Is a Science

OUR QUEST FOR PERFECT PRODUCE

Fruits piled in baskets. Vegetables stacked in crates. Melons and ears of corn cracked open to show freshness. Bugs buzzing around in the sun. Wait. Bugs? Sun?

> **Food Truth**
>
> Food is an amazing science from farm to table.

If you've ever shopped for food in a less developed country, you likely have visited an outdoor market. There is no refrigeration, no USDA or FDA, and little regulation on how food can be sold. In Egypt, I saw raw meat hanging next to tomatoes, with flies on both. In Mexico, I admired beautiful melons split open to taste, but wondered about the many hands that had been in the melon. In South Africa, there were meats laid out beside cheeses, next to corn in a glass case as the vendor waved away bugs with his hand.

In contrast, stores in the United Kingdom, Canada, the United States, and Australia invest millions in food presentation—and marketing. In the United States we seek "perfect produce" and turn away from anything with a blemish. Studies show that freshness consistently ranks as a priority, so it's interesting to consider where freshness begins as a green growing plant and ends as a rotten refrigerator mess.

The big questions and food myths:

- *How do I really know what is fresh?*
- *If it's natural, isn't it fresh?*

GROWING AND HARVESTING FRESHNESS

Long before a vegetable is ever in your grocery cart, it is a seed. A seed that is planted in the ground at the right time in the right conditions that grows into a plant. The plant requires nutrients and protection from predators (bugs, fungus, weeds) to reach reproductive stage.

After the plant pollinates, it bears fruit (which is the term referred to all veggies and fruits) either above or below the ground. The fruit then requires protection from predators, which now includes wildlife (and their waste). If all of these steps are successful, the fruit grows and produce is harvested. Harvest requires great care, as ripe produce is fragile. That care includes the right equipment, temperature, and timing. Then the produce is trucked off the farm.

Freshness begins on the farm, but it certainly isn't where it ends. Temperature reigns as king of vegetables—it is the defining factor for a "fresh" product that looks and tastes good and that lasts in your refrigerator.

TEMPERATURE IS KING

California farmer Ryan Van Groningen talks more about the farm's role in producing and harvesting sweet corn as the best science they apply to freshness.

"To be honest, a grower does not have full control of how fresh sweet corn is at the grocery store. We only play a small part in the process. We purchase and plant seed that is sweet corn, not field corn that would be used for animal feed.

"We harvest daily to keep product fresh, and sweet corn is very sensitive to warmer temperatures so it is extremely important to cool sweet corn down to 32 to 34 degrees Fahrenheit as soon as possible after harvest. When sweet corn pulp temperatures are above that level, sugars in the kernels begin to turn to starch.

"Besides temperature, sweet corn will also begin turning sugars into starch over time. As you can tell, the grocery store has a large part in keeping sweet corn fresh by rotating stock quickly and by not breaking the cold chain," he explained.

That also means that if you buy your veggies at the store on an 80-degree day and decide to run two hours of errands before you get home, your veggies aren't going to last as long. They like to keep the "cold chain" going, even in your home—that's the science in freshness.

Rousseau Farming Company, who grows more than 20 types of vegetables and has been continuously ranked as a top 10 Southwest farm for over 15 years, agrees temperature after harvest is critical to freshness. "Cooling is the single most important element to keep produce fresh and of high quality. How quickly it's cooled and if it's cooled to the right temperature is the most important item in preserving freshness."

GROWING FRESHNESS FROM THE GROUND UP

A standby vegetable you can count on to remain fresh in the pantry for a long time is the potato, thanks to the science in growing these tubers. It seems potatoes have gotten a bad rap because of French fries and chips; potatoes actually are an amazing source of potassium and are important to heart health when you keep them out of the fryer.

Such was pointed out to me by a man very passionate about potatoes: John Halverson of Black Gold Farms in North Dakota. They farm across 10 states and have about 35,000 acres of potatoes, sweet potatoes, corn, wheat, and soybeans.

John, along with his brother, sister, and dad, own Black Gold Farms, and they are one of the largest chip suppliers in the United States. Black Gold also sells sweet potatoes and red potatoes to large retailers throughout the country.

When I asked John how such a large operation with 200 employees could be a family farm, he was quick to respond: "We are absolutely a family farm and have been since 1928. It's what we do. The Halverson family still goes and plays in the dirt."

The best preservative for a table potato is a tough skin, accomplished through the science of farming. John described the complex business of growing potatoes across 11 farms, starting with the seed potato. "Potatoes take a whole lot of seed, about an average of about 2,500 pounds per acre, depending on the variety and region. The seed is stored 36 to 38 degrees Fahrenheit, to keep it dormant, and then a machine cuts the seed potato into 2.2-ounce pieces." The seeds are treated with a fir bark material to help their wounds heal, piled on the ground with blown air to warm them up, and then planted several days later.

"Before planting, if there are nematodes present, the soil is fumigated in the south to kill nematodes that like to clog up the root system, though that's not always necessary. Potash is applied to fields beforehand, then about 200 to 350 pounds of nitrogen is put on per acre throughout the season in six or seven different applications—about 20 percent less than they used to. At planting, starter fertilizer (phosphate and zinc), fungicide, and insecticide to keep leaf hopper and Colorado beetle away for 90 to 100 days, to minimize spraying the plants, are all put into the ground with the seed potato."

John went on to explain their planter captures real-time data and they're collaborating with John Deere to use the information to improve sustainability. The data is collected on every farm and he monitors the numbers remotely; he can see a screen of what's being planted in Winamac, Indiana, while he is sitting in his office in Missouri.

"There's nothing that is ever perfect, as seeds change, field conditions change, weather changes, etc. The data allows us to see this transparently and make adjustments as necessary. The potato is fantastic at converting energy into food," John explained.

It can take potatoes 50 days to come out of the ground because the seeds aren't as physiologically aged as seeds you may plant in your garden. However, when they do come up, potatoes grow fast—they go from peeking through the soil to covering the ground in two or three weeks.

Water is an important part of growing healthy potatoes, but they are a very sustainable crop. Black Gold Farms uses center pivot irrigation (the kind that makes circles) to irrigate often, but with a lesser amount of water than row crops.

Herbicides are used as needed, with one to three applications during the growing season to minimize weeds because they can compete with and weaken potato plants, though there are not a lot of herbicides approved for use in this crop. Once potatoes are a foot tall, fungicides start to protect the plants from late blight and other diseases. It is this blight that caused the Irish potato famine, as it destroys the leaf and tubers. If the crop becomes infected with late blight, the potato plants have to be killed as soon as possible and harvested immediately.

Tissue samples of potatoes are taken throughout the season to check the nutrient level of the plants to ensure the crop is in the best condition possible. The irrigation water is also checked regularly for *E. coli*. And potatoes also are tested for residues.

"Our potato has been respected its entire life. Anything the government says is in rules, that's the way it has been treated. Since it's not a big crop, with respect to acres in the United States, there's not a lot of products developed for potatoes. They always err on the side of caution with approved chemistries for potato and make longer pre-harvest intervals."

Black Gold Farms believes in label integrity and maintains a zero-tolerance policy for using products "off label" (at different rates or mixtures than those approved by the EPA). "The truth is easy to defend," John said as he explained why they shut down a chip plant in Texas. "We needed to harvest two days earlier than what was labeled for grass herbicide that was applied. We made the decision to not deliver them to the plant and maintain our label integrity."

Every step of the way is GLOBAL G.A.P. certified, whether it's a sweet potato, table potato, or chip potato. After potatoes are harvested, they are then trucked off to be cooled and washed, put in citric acid (like an orange juice) so the potatoes don't turn dark, and then get Selectrocide sprayed on them to kill any bacteria and prevent decay.

PRESERVATION AT PROCESSING AND PACKAGING

Selectrocide is a food-grade antibacterial used for food safety and is commonly used in produce. It is registered with the EPA and the Organic Review Material

Institute (ORMI), and it's approved by the FDA. Chlorine dioxide, the active ingredient in Selectrocide is used for water treatment, cleaning fruit and vegetables, and food storage facilities, according to EnviroPure USA.

Treating produce with products like Selectrocide before packaging neutralizes any harmful pathogens that may be present, such as *Salmonella* or *E. coli*. The use of these sanitizers is required by federal regulation before produce can be sold. Gas, such as carbon dioxide, is also used to fill produce packages to stop the growth of microbes.

Why all the science in protecting freshness? A series of outbreaks and product recalls, such as a 2006 *E. coli* outbreak in fresh spinach that resulted in over 270 hospitalizations and three deaths. Unfortunately, where produce grows, bacteria go, particularly when wildlife are involved.

Research is being conducted to further improve produce freshness and safety by Michigan State University, Ohio State University, and Rutgers University, through a $2 million grant from the USDA. "After being treated with sanitizers, many products are packaged under various atmospheres and exposed to fluctuating temperature conditions, which can increase the chances that they become contaminated or lose their freshness. Our findings will be built into the USDA's risk assessment program to improve food safety."[54]

20. What's Growing in Your Veggie Drawer?

THE EYES OF HUNGER

Visiting South Africa is a memory I'll carry for the rest of my life, especially the eyes of hungry children. Children who live in squatters' camps by the millions. Children who live in shacks that make a dog house look like a condominium. Children who play next to bootlegged raw electrical lines. Children who don't care about the politics of food, but only where they can get their next meal.

> **Food Truth**
>
> The answer to food waste is hidden in your refrigerator.

I've seen those same eyes in Egypt from children begging. And in the Ukraine shortly after communism fell. Then back in Indiana when my daughter started school and had hungry classmates.

The debate we have around food in developed countries is a very privileged one. Yet, even in the United States, one in six people go hungry. That number rises globally. Yet today it is more righteous to debate the politics of food than the very real problem of hunger.

What's the answer to food insecurity and hunger? It is a multifaceted answer, part of which has to be solving food waste in this country.

The big questions and food myths:

- *Is food waste really a problem?*
- *How am I supposed to fix such a major problem?*

FORTY PERCENT OF OUR FOOD IS WASTED

Americans throw away 40 percent of the country's food supply. Fresh fruits and vegetables account for 22 percent of total food loss from retail, restaurants, and household. Processed fruits and vegetables add another 8 percent—nearly one-third the total food wasted. That's a whole lot of smelly fruits and veggies![55]

I'm just as guilty as anyone—my veggies sometimes ferment into lettuce silage, and fruit goes unnoticed in the back of the refrigerator until it is a pile of brown mush. How does your refrigerator look?

Most waste happens at a consumer level. We let food go bad in the fridge or misunderstand the meaning of expiration dates and throw away food before it's actually expired. But some waste happens at the production and retail levels—produce that isn't perfect may not be harvested on the farm, and restaurants and grocery stores toss food before it's spoiled to make room for new shipments.

The USDA and EPA announced the first-ever food waste reduction goal for the United States in 2015, calling for a 50 percent reduction by 2030. Food is the single biggest contributor to landfills today: 133 billion pounds of it end up in dumpsters each year in America.[56]

We trash about $162 billion worth of food across the nation, which uses up about 25 percent of the U.S. water supply and produces 33 million cars' worth of greenhouse gases annually. When in landfills, food waste releases methane, a greenhouse gas. Yet, one in six Americans live in food insecurity, and many of those have little access to produce.[57]

FARMERS MINIMIZING FOOD WASTE

At the announcement of the food waste reduction initiative, then USDA secretary Tom Vilsack said, "The United States enjoys the most productive and abundant food supply on earth, but too much of this food goes to waste. Our new reduction goal demonstrates America's leadership on a global level in getting wholesome food to people who need it, protecting our natural resources, cutting environmental pollution, and promoting innovative approaches for reducing food loss and waste."

Farmers are trying to do their part. It's not a perfect system, and waste needs to be reduced across agriculture, but many farms and ranches use every single product they can, creating a recycling program many cities would admire. If food-grade products don't meet standards, they become animal feed. If products can't be fed to animals, they're used as fertilizers.

When asked about food waste, Ryan Van Groningen said, "We are huge proponents of the food bank. Anything that will not meet grade goes to the food bank. We also have begun juicing which allows us to use more off-grade product for juicing or concentrate. The only product we throw away is product that is broken, cracked, etc., because of food safety concerns."

Likewise, the Schmidts in Maryland had problems with some of their green beans speckling from a rain right before harvest, so they donated them to the Maryland Food Bank. The Rousseaus in Arizona say they aim to harvest all food off of the farm, but inevitably there is usually some small quality issue or pest problem that makes that more difficult. If individuals weren't so concerned with cosmetic problems in their produce, more food would make it into the marketplace.

Produce discarded by retailers can also be used in animal feed rather than being put in a landfill, like the scrap produce used by the Kuehnerts in Indiana to feed their dairy cattle. It's not uncommon for livestock farmers living near a processing or retail center to recycle "waste" food products for animal feed.

What Role Can You Play in Reducing Food Waste?

Limit your trips to the store, store your produce properly, know expiration timelines, freeze what you can't use soon, and use common sense on what's good or not.

21. A Love of Playing in the Soil

A RELATIONSHIP WITH THE LAND

A dad of six who sells at three different farmers' markets and drives a grocery store delivery truck. Meet Tyson Roberts, a vegetable grower just outside of Salt Lake City, Utah—a man who wears many hats. When asked why he farms, he quickly responds, "It's a relationship with the land, with the soil. It's how I was raised and how I want my kids to be raised. It's a family thing. Our land has been in our family for 150 years."

> **Food Truth**
> Soil is a farm's greatest asset.

Tyson is proud that his 15-year-old daughter and 12-year-old son are already involved in helping manage the farm's presence at an urban farmers' market. He talks about life lessons that he learned on the farm, lessons he hopes to pass on to his children.

The farm raises sweet corn, potatoes, popcorn, garlic, sweet potatoes, onions, cucumbers, peppers, and tomatoes—he likes to say his farm grows "anything you need for salsa." His family has a small farm in an area that's growing more houses, with land prices around $100,000 an acre.

Roberts Family Farms have carved out a niche, selling 70 percent of their products retail (at farmers' markets or on the honor system at the farm stand) and 30 percent at a local grocery store or through a produce buyer. They raise small quantities of many vegetable crops and try something new every few years. This year it's kale, grown in greenhouses with tomatoes.

Their business is a great example of how all of us owe our existence to soil—and the nutrition that comes forth when water is added to the earth.

The big questions and food myths:

- *Why does dirt matter?*
- *Don't farmers care more about profit than the land?*
- *How do you grow vegetables?*

SOIL IS NOT DIRT

These questions are those the Roberts family hears at the farmers' markets about soil. They are careful to talk about how they live on the land, care for the land, and their family eats from the land. They are equally as careful to tell people they do not farm organically—and why.

"If you treat the soil right, it will return for you what you invest in it," Tyson insists. He partners with his neighbor, who has a small plot of organic greens (spinach, kale, and collard), and sees no difference in the soil health. There is no doubt the 15 acres adjacent to his home hold a special place in his heart. "It's been there for 150 years in my family, I want it to be just as good in the next 150 years."

Soil is not dirt. Soil is the foundation of all food production.

Crop rotation is critical for soil management when growing vegetables. Some crops, like tomatoes, use a lot of nutrients, so rotation protects the soil from having too many nutrients taken up by plants. It's also logical to rotate because certain types of ground are not suited to growing different crops. If you plant a product in the wrong soil type, it is susceptible to different diseases, increases pressure from weeds, and you'll end up spending a whole lot more on inputs (the products to provide nutrients or combat diseases).

In other words, farmers growing crops need to be soil scientists. It's especially true for those planting a variety of crops like vegetables; the farmer has to know their soil type and what they are planting. Soil can change dramatically in half a mile. Some ground is sandier, some is heavier. Potatoes and tomatoes are in the same family so they can't be planted annually right after each other. Research is required to know which rotations (the order crops are planted in) result in more problems with diseases in the plants.

Soil testing is done in the spring before planting and again in the fall so farmers can compare what winter does with the soil. Some fields require nitrogen, but the amount, timing, and application differ based upon crop, soil, and time of year. The soil in the other fields requires potassium and phosphate, which is plowed into the root zone. Yet another specific area may require iron. Soil health has a lot of moving pieces to put together.

Biomass, usually in the form of leftover plants (e.g., wheat straw or corn stalk), provides the most returns. "Soil is healthier today than when I started farming. We're putting a lot more back into the soil. We are much more conscientious of the soil," Tyson says.

Healthy soil grows more food. Healthy soil requires fewer inputs. Healthy soil preserves generations of farmers. Healthy soil requires less water. Healthy soil just makes sense for farmers.

WEED CONTROL

Like larger farmers, Tyson uses weed control to minimize the amount of weeds they have to manually handle or have to interfere with the harvest. "We have done this to control weeds for as long I can remember."

Once the seeds are in, he scouts daily for five days after planting to spray weed control in the onion field right before plants emerge. "Onions are the crop that takes the most herbicide because harvest is a nightmare if there is a weed problem. Weeds plug up harvest machines and loading machines by tangling in the chains."

Different vegetables have different bug issues treated in different ways. "Crop rotation helps with bugs—if we plant a half mile away there won't be the bug pressure." In other words, planting peppers where onions were last year can reduce the insects that eat peppers.

Tyson drives to his different fields every Monday to "scout" the different crops to look for specific problems, such as insects. "A lot of scouting one day of the week will tell us priorities for the rest of the week. I use a notebook and different apps on my phone to track what's in each field. I use Google Keep as an ongoing checklist, and also use it as my grocery list. A lot of my records are digital."

Many of their farmers' market customers ask if they use pesticides. Tyson confirms they do, but emphasizes integrated pest management (IPM). "We don't want to use too many pesticides because they're expensive."

Farmers apply a lot of science and expertise to caring for their land to raise food, whether on 50 acres in Utah or 5,000 acres in Arizona. Nurturing the soil is key to their existence—and ours. Healthy soil grows healthy food for you.

Table 4   Vegetable Food Truths

Food Myth	Food Truth
Farmers are profiting from the increase in food price.	**Food Truth 7: Food costs are a shared concern.** A farmer receives less than 15 cents from each dollar you spend on food. They do everything they can to reduce costs while raising safe food—and they are consuming it, too!
Chemicals on vegetables are poisoning your family.	**Food Truth 10: Chemicals are naturally in food and are needed to protect it.** Where vegetables grow, pests go. Tomatoes without worms and potatoes without rot require chemicals. And chemicals aren't all bad—vegetables are actually producing their own.
Fresh veggies require no intervention.	**Food Truth 13: Food is an amazing science from farm to table.** Less-than-perfect food is often discarded, so the science of preserving produce is critical to avoid the vegetable graveyard.
Grocery stores and restaurants need to solve food waste.	**Food Truth 14: The answer to food waste is hidden in your refrigerator.** Food that is thrown out both at home and on the farm—in the search for the perfect pepper—is the largest contributor to food waste.
Farmers destroy soil in the interest of profits.	**Food Truth 15: Soil is a farm's greatest asset.** Protecting the soil for future crops—and generations—is a priority for people working the land.

Part V: Meats

Pretty red barns, cute talking animals, and farmers in overalls make for a good book and movie, as long as you realize they're fiction. An inside look from farmers and ranchers on how animals are raised, why many farms are larger, and a comparison of different types of animal care to help you feel good about the protein your family gets from the meat case.

"Nature is cruel, but we don't have to be."

—Temple Grandin

22. The Mayhem of Meat. Why Isn't Farming Like *Charlotte's Web?*

THE BEATING OF PRINCESS

My friend Kelly, who milks my cows, called me on a sticky 90-degree day in August, her normally calm voice distressed. "I just found Princess down in the pasture. Can you come help?" Princess was one of the cows descended from Perfect (see the dairy case story).

> **Food Truth**
>
> Animal welfare is an hourly concern on farms and ranches.

As I raced over to the pasture, I saw Princess lying stretched out. She appeared to have been down (unable to stand) for several hours in the sun and heat. She was laboring to breathe.

Kelly hurried off to the barn to get the tractor. What I had to do keep Princess' heart pumping was not pretty. This required me smacking her across the face and kneeing her chest as hard as my human weight could muster. Before you judge me, consider the shock it takes to keep a human heart going. A physician often cracks ribs while giving chest compressions. Multiply that force by 10.

Kelly returned with the heavy equipment; we got Princess up by putting a metal device known as a hip lift around her hips. Kelly raised the lift with the tractor, and I provided leverage on the halter so Princess could stand.

As we waited for her to become steady enough to walk, we talked about how terrible the incident would look on video if captured by animal rights activists. We helped Princess back to the barn, with Kelly carefully driving the tractor and the hip lifts holding Princess up, as I kept her steady on the halter. It was not a pretty scene; urine was pouring out of the cow and there was manure everywhere—cows don't use bedpans.

Is this an image I want on camera? I think not. Not because I have anything to hide, and not because I abuse animals, but because few people would have the context of how we were focused on animal welfare. It would look terrible on the nightly news and be incorrectly labeled as animal abuse.

Yet the cow lived and did not suffer needlessly because two women cared enough to do some ugly things in the interest of animal care. Sometimes drastic measures are necessary to save a life.

Farming often isn't a pretty business. There is mud, manure, blood, and sweat. Context matters.

The big questions and food myths:

- *How are farm animals really treated behind closed doors?*
- *Do farmers care more about money or doing the right thing for their animals?*
- *Should I feel guilty that animals die so I eat?*

IT IS NOT AN OXYMORON TO RAISE ANIMALS FOR FOOD AND TREAT THEM WITH RESPECT

Yes, animals die so we can eat—that is the animal's purpose. Farmers raise animals because they care deeply for animals; it's not simply profit driven. Yes, farmers and ranchers derive their income from animals, but the work required 365 days a year is driven by a concern for animals.

I go to the barn to be sure my animals have food and water because I care about their well-being on an ethical level. It is the right thing to do. Although there are some farmers and ranchers who do not operate that way, I've met very few who do not put the care of their animals first. Animal care comes before their own meal, family event, or fun with friends. Not because of money, but because it is the right thing to do.

Do farmers dehorn, trim teeth, manage beaks, and castrate animals? Yes. Do farmers do these things to pad their pockets with cash? No. Are there improvements that could be made? Sure, that's called progress—which is what the agricultural community strives for.

However, all of these practices are designed to protect the animals from themselves—and protect the people who are handling the animals. It is not an oxymoron to raise animals for food and treat them with respect.

Animals can be cruel. They can destroy each other and hurt a human faster than you can imagine. Perhaps not what you want to think about as you enjoy chicken wings, cheeseburgers, or pork chops, yet really important in the conversation around animal welfare.

Why? Because it's essential to understand animal behavior if you want to discuss animal welfare.

BACON BULLIES

Pigs are omnivores—they like meat and plants. Apologies for being blunt, but they'll eat each other if given the chance. Pigs are known for targeting a lame or weaker animal and then biting it. The trimming of eye teeth in piglets helps reduce injury, as does the docking of their tails. It may sound cruel, but it's actually being kind to the animal. You see, hogs will actually grab each other by their curly tails and begin gnawing if the tails are not trimmed.

Wanda Patsche, grandma to six and a swine farmer with her husband Chuck in the rolling hills of southern Minnesota, sums up pig temperaments. "I wish people could experience the things we experience. I wish they could see the fights sows have, which are a natural response to their innate social hierarchy that determines who is the 'king' sow.

"They fight until they injure each other. They bite body parts including ears, snouts, and legs. And sometimes these injuries are lethal. I wish people could hear the ear-piercing screams we hear when a sow is attacking another. No, we don't rush to grab our phones to videotape the pig attacks. Instead, we attempt to break up the fights, assess and care for the injuries, all while hoping not to be injured ourselves."

The battle for pecking order starts immediately after birth as the piglets are fighting to nurse.

Wanda points out, "Piglets screech and squeal whenever their feet are off the ground. Every time. They hardly even notice when their tails and teeth are trimmed; they immediately go back to nursing when they're put back with their momma sow. The trimming is done with hand tools, and there's no pulling involved. Veterinarians agree these are the right practices so the pigs don't get scratched up."

The farm tried not trimming the piglets' teeth for a while, but the momma sows were in pain—they'd jump up from being bitten while nursing. If you've ever breastfeed a child with teeth, you can appreciate a sow's predicament.

RAISING A HEALTHY PIG

Wanda lives in the sixth largest hog-producing county in the United States. The winters are brutal—they went through three major blizzards last winter. "All of our pigs are now raised indoors, which is very typical of the area due to our extreme temperatures. Having the pigs in barns protects them from the cold, keeps them away from predators, and gives the pigs clean air and water 24 hours per day. Barns also protect the pigs from birds transmitting virus and disease and humans from getting trichinosis.

"It used to be we worried about keeping pigs alive when it stormed; there was snow over the waterer, their bedding was always wet, and getting feed to them was tough. Now we can focus on how to better care for the animal and how to feed them more scientifically."

Disease management is a big deal on a farm—similar to the way it would be at a daycare. This is why barns are closed; not because farmers want to keep secrets, but in the interest of keeping their animals healthy. "When one pig is sick, the others can be mean. They pick on it non-stop. The pig has to be pulled out of the pen and put into a hospital," said Wanda.

Animal welfare is not just a catchphrase on farms or ranches. It is a reality. Every day. No matter how cold or hot.

Animals are naturally hunters and fighters. It's called survival of the fittest. Consider the lion hunting a gazelle in South Africa, the fight of alley cats, or how a bear rips a deer to shreds. None are particularly pleasant, but all are instinctual behaviors.

The same instinctual behaviors exist in farm animals. It is the job of the farmer and rancher to manage the animals in their care, to ensure animal welfare through environment and best practices.

Wanda pointed out, "It's a lot of hard work and you have to have the passion for this. If you don't have that, you won't last long. They definitely test you. Our complete focus is to raise the healthiest pig we can. It's the right thing to do, and we can only sell healthy pigs; our contractor will not take a pig with a bloodied tail or one that is limping. The main focus we have every single day is to raise a healthy pig."

PROTECTING ANIMALS FROM EACH OTHER

Poultry are also omnivores. They like meat, as well as grains. Their beaks are managed because they are cruel to each other when they reach adolescence. They will peck each other to death. So beak management is a common practice in male turkeys, which involves holding up a pullet (baby turkey) and filing or lasering the beak. If this photo was shared across Instagram and taken out of context, you may perceive that the turkeys are being tortured. Again, context matters. Beaks are managed to protect the birds from each other.

The castration of cattle and hogs is another practice commonly questioned. Why castrate? Males with their testicles are aggressive. I don't mean aggressive like football players wanting to tackle each other; I mean "hide-in-a-dark-alley and flip you into the air" aggressive. I never went in the bull pen without protection. Seeing bulls flip people into the air or pummel a full-grown man into the ground taught me to never turn my back on them.

Besides the safety factor, meat from intact male animals (those that have not been castrated and still have testicles) is often tough and off-flavor. As such, the vast majority of beef and pork comes from steers and barrows (male cattle and pigs that have been castrated).

There has been a loud call for transparency about what farmers and ranchers are doing to animals. Do farmers or ranchers value an animal's life the same as the rest of society? Yes, farmers and ranchers actually place more value on the animals because of the ongoing care they give them so the animals can provide food for humans. That is honorable; eating meat should not evoke guilt. And proper animal care is the right thing to do for the animal *and* any farm business—it's not an either-or situation.

Transparent animal welfare involves practices that appear really ugly when taken out of context. It protects the animals from themselves and keeps people safe. While not pretty, animals welfare practices are done for the right reason by people who best know animals—farmers, ranchers, and veterinarians.

23. Are Antibiotics Awful?

MOTHERS STANDING IN JUDGMENT

While I was at a meeting for farm women, we took a tour of a dairy farm and spent some time looking at calf care. Raising healthy "babies" (calves, piglets, etc.) is an area women are often charged with on the farm—and excel at it—with a mothering instinct that translates to animal care instincts. And there can be plenty of judgment involved.

> **Food Truth**
> Antibiotics have benefits.

"Did you see those calves? I don't think they're feeding them right," was the first whisper I heard from one woman as we walked among the calves. "I think they need to be treated—I would give them electrolytes" was the next comment. There were a couple of calves that weren't feeling their best, and the longer we were in the calf area, the more negative comments I heard from the women about poor calf care. I had to quietly smile as I stood back and watched these women, normally very kind and generous, make judgmental statements about what they would be doing to help the calves.

You see, each woman there took calf care very personally. When our animals are sick, we are in distress. All the momma-bear tendencies show up. Not because we are profit driven, but because having healthy calves, piglets, or chicks is personal. And we want to use the tools we know will treat sickness, which includes antibiotics. Keeping the babies healthy is important!

The big questions and food myths:

- *Are there antibiotics in meat?*
- *Are antibiotics given to overcome mistreatment of animals in poor environments?*
- *Is antibiotic use in farm animals creating resistance in humans?*

TESTED EQUALS TRUSTED: RESIDUE VERSUS RESISTANCE

Did you know every food product must be technically free of antibiotic residue? It has been so since the 1950s, when the FDA banned all violative antibiotic residues in finished food products. Farmers have to follow requirements for withdrawal times—the time it takes for antibiotics to work their way out of an animal's system before the animal is allowed to be slaughtered. These requirements protect food against residue.

The late Dr. Scott Hurd, former deputy undersecretary for food safety at the USDA, a veterinarian, and professor at Iowa State University, showed there is a one in a billion chance of treatment failure from antibiotic resistances related to the use of common animal antibiotics. One in a billion!

"Due to farmers following appropriate withdrawal times, there are very few violations. In fact in the last three years of USDA testing no broiler chickens have been found with violative residues for the scheduled (random) sampling. For beef only two violations out of 1,600 samples were found and only three out of 2,200 from market hogs. Note that antibiotics are not toxins, they are useful and very safe products used by us all."[58]

"An antibiotic is a chemical substance, produced by microorganisms, which has the capacity to inhibit the growth of and even to destroy bacteria and other microorganisms," according to the pure definition of an antibiotic, still used in textbooks today, written in 1947 by Dr. Waksman.[59]

Meat is tested for antibiotic residue. There are maximum levels, measured in trace amounts, determined by the National Residue Program. The USDA's Food Safety and Inspection Service (FSIS) works with the EPA and FDA to test for a variety of residues such as antibiotics, pesticides, and environmental toxins under the National Residue Program.[60]

Resistance is different from residue—they are not related. Resistance means an antibiotic is no longer as effective. Resistance is also measured and reported through the National Antimicrobial Resistance Monitoring System.

Basically, resistance refers to one microbe (e.g., bacteria) no longer having the power it once did over another microbe. In other words, antibiosis is the bullying of one bacterium over another. Today's bacteria are becoming bigger bullies by producing more substances to kill other bacteria—there is an increasing number evolving in order to survive, becoming resistant to antibiotics.

DO WE GIVE HUMAN DRUGS TO ANIMALS?

FDA statistics show 87 percent of antibiotics used in animals is either never or very rarely used in human medicine. An animal is not human. An animal—even your dog and cat—is treated different medically than a human. But an animal needs antibiotics if it is sick from bacteria. Antibiotics can be beneficial.[61]

According to the 2013 IMS Institute for Healthcare report on human health, "The misuse of antibiotics contributes to antimicrobial resistance and an estimated $34 billion each year in avoidable inpatient care costs. An additional $1 billion is spent on about 31 million inappropriate antibiotic prescriptions that are dispensed each year, typically for viral infections. There are encouraging signs that efforts to drive responsible antibiotics use are paying off, particularly in the declining number of prescriptions for the common cold and flu—viral infections that do not respond to antibiotics."[62]

Dr. Richard Raymond is the former undersecretary for food safety with the U.S. Department of Agriculture. He graduated from the University of Nebraska Medical School with distinction and had long-time family practices in Nebraska, where he also served as that state's chief medical officer. He has written a great deal about antibiotics and food animals, including "Lies, Damn Lies and Statistics" in *Food Safety News*:[63]

Antibiotics critical to human health include the cephalosporin and the fluoroquinolone classes. These two classes of antibiotics made up 24 percent of all human antibiotics sold in 2009, but combined, they only represented 0.3 percent of all antibiotics sold for use in animal health.

The reason for this disparity is that the FDA has already used its regulatory authority to limit these two categories of antibiotics to full therapeutic use to treat disease states in animals, limiting bacterial exposure to these antibiotics of critical importance to human health.

So when you read a report funded by the Pew Charitable Trust, or Consumers Union, stating that they found Salmonella sp. bacteria resistant to Cipro (a fluoroquinolone), where do you think that resistance came from? From the 11,000 kilograms used in animals, or from the 304,741 kilograms prescribed to treat humans?

Speaking of resistance in bacteria, penicillin was discovered in 1943; by 1950, just 7 short years later, 40 percent of all Staph isolates from U.S. hospital intensive care units were resistant to penicillin. By 1960 that number was 80 percent.

Methicillin was discovered in 1959. In 1960 the first case of methicillin-resistant *Staphylococcus aureus* (MRSA) was found in England. Confined Animal Feeding Operations (CAFOs) did not contribute to this rapidly developing resistance. Human use did.

PORK CHOPS, BACON, AND MEDICATION?

Chris Chinn is a mom of two married to her high school sweetheart, and they dream of their two teenagers becoming the sixth generation to farm in Missouri. She shares her perspective on how antibiotics are used on their hog farm, where they have 1,600 sows:

On our farm, it's normal for us to have entire groups of pigs that never have had any antibiotics when they go to market. Yes, you read that correctly. I know this is not what you see on the Internet about how farmers use antibiotics. It seems everywhere you look you can read or hear a very different story. I'm here to tell you this is a myth.

I like to explain our antibiotic use like this: our hogs do not carry health insurance and all medications are expensive. We cannot afford to use antibiotics unless absolutely necessary to improve the quality of health for our animals. And we always use antibiotics under the guidance of our veterinarian. He decides what medication will be used when necessary and what dose will be used.

We have a healthcare plan for our hogs that is designed by our veterinarian. This means when we detect a hog might be sick or that a hog isn't behaving normally, we call in our veterinarian and follow his advice in how to protect that animal and keep it healthy.

Antibiotics are just one of the tools we have in our tool box; we don't rely on them as part of our daily care plan. On our farm, we work hard to prevent problems from occurring, that's why we are so strict about protecting our hogs' environment. We wash and disinfect our barns on a routine basis for prevention. Our sow barns are washed weekly (these barns house the adult females that will give birth to piglets). And each sow (adult female that has given birth before) is bathed before going to the farrowing barn where they will give birth. Our gilts are also bathed before farrowing—a gilt is a female hog that has not given birth before. We do this to prevent infection during the birthing process and it also relaxes the sow or gilt and helps keep them comfortable. We also wash and sanitize our nursery barns and finisher barns before every new group of pigs arrive to the barn.

We use very, very little antibiotics because we prevent problems from occurring. By keeping our hogs indoors in a climate-controlled barn, we eliminated the biggest threats to our hogs' health, and thus decrease the need for antibiotics. For example, we prevent fighting between our sows by using independent maternity pens. Fighting results in injuries. These injuries used to be one of the main reasons we had to use antibiotics on our farm. We have also decreased the need for antibiotics on our farm by keeping our hogs away from predators and wildlife that spread disease.

We are required to log all antibiotic use on our farm. This means if we use an antibiotic on a pig or a sow, we have to record the date, medication given, dose, and withdrawal length. We are audited by the plant that purchases our hogs, and they inspect these records a couple times a year. They also review my feed records to see what we feed our hogs. They want to make sure they are purchasing a healthy hog from me. But this isn't why we keep these records. We keep these records for our own benefit as well; my kids and I eat the same pork I sell for other families to serve on their dinner tables. I love my two kids more than anything in this world. I don't want to feed my kids anything that isn't safe to eat. I am a mom, this is one of the most important jobs I will ever have and I take that responsibility very seriously.

So, as you can see, it doesn't make any sense for me to misuse antibiotics on my farm, nor would I ever choose to. I simply stand to lose too much if I don't use them correctly.

She's not in the minority to have this mindset. Imagine you own a business with a million dollars invested in the equipment, services, inputs, and infrastructure. You have a contract to sell all of your product. One mistake is made, and all of your product is tainted—the buyer will no longer take your product. That is the exact reality of farming and ranching—protocols are followed or you lose your business.

STEAK ON A HEALTHY HOOF

Dusty Hahn is a fifth-generation rancher out in Montana—both sides of his family have operated ranches continuously for 100 years. Hahn's Ranch is a family ranching corporation located on the Missouri River in Townsend. The family business is a diversified operation that includes cow/calf farming, cattle feeding (a feedlot), trucking, and ag service enterprises.

There are currently four generations on the Hahn ranch. Dusty posted this on Facebook, along with a picture of one of his steers (a castrated male), explaining how and why he treats his beef cattle with antibiotics.

This is a steer calf that came to my feedlot a couple days ago. His official ID is 0609, because that is his mother's ear tag number. His momma called him "Moo," but I don't speak cow, so his nickname is Dave.

Anyway, it seems Dave contracted foot rot. He got it out on the open range. It's nasty stuff. Like athlete's foot on steroids. It's a bacterial infection. Its scientific name is infectious pododermatitis. Look it up. The definition includes phrases like: 'It is extremely painful and contagious,' and, 'It can be treated with a series of medications, but if not treated, the whole herd can become infected.'

I don't like the sounds of any of that! But luckily, I'm an expert at treating foot rot. So, I captured young Dave in the head catch. He didn't like it much, but anything has to be better than suffering from this foot rot. Luckily, since foot rot is a bacterial infection, I have a product called oxytetracycline that is FDA approved for the treatment of foot rot. The product I use is called Bio-Mycin 200. It has an approved dosage amount, which is conveniently located on the label. So, since Dave weighs 550#, he gets 25 milliliters of antibiotic. But, according to Beef Quality Assurance (BQA) guidelines, he can't have more than 10 milliliters of antibiotic in any injection site. Furthermore, Bio-Mycin is labeled, and again approved by the FDA, for administration by intramuscular (in the muscle tissue), subcutaneous (under the skin, between skin and muscle tissue), or intravenous (in a vein, directly into the blood stream) injection. Since I'm a BQA guy, I always opt for the sub Q (under the skin) route whenever possible so the muscle isn't damaged.

Dave got three injections of about eight milliliters of Oxytet under his skin in the neck area. No antibiotic went into the muscle tissue, and even if it did, Dave's going to be living with me for the next 150 days. The withdrawal period on Oxytet is a whopping 28 days. Which means that his system will clear the antibiotic out in a MONTH! That means Dave will be drug-free for over four months when he leaves my ranch!

I could have chosen not to help Dave out, but that just seems WRONG! Plus, since foot rot is extremely contagious, I would just as soon not have his counterparts contracting it, too. I could post another video in 10 days or 2 weeks, but I guarantee that Dave will not be limping, will not be in pain, and will be as healthy as all his buddies.

That is why I will continue to use antibiotics responsibly and judiciously at my ranch.

Note the FDA states that animals treated with antibiotics are not allowed to be butchered for a specific period of time after treatment. Meat is tested throughout the butchering process and is disposed of if a sample is found to have any trace of antibiotics, at the cost of the producer.

Each food sector has penalties in place for cheaters. In today's robust testing environment, cheaters get caught. Therefore, there is no value in cheating, and it proves the system works.

HEALTHY GUTS

One of the ways cattle are kept healthy is by protecting their gut health through products called ionophores. The benefit is similar to that of probiotics used by humans to promote "good" bacteria. But ionophores are classified as antibiotics in the United States—though not in the European Union—and are the reason why there is a difference in food label claims between the EU and the United States. Ionophores work against the bad bacteria in the rumen of a cow and hind-gut in a pig to favor those bacteria aiding in digestion and to inhibit bad bacteria. That's a win for food safety and keeping animals healthier; ionophores are diges-tive aids to help animals better use their good bugs. They're not effective in human medicine and have no human application, but are approved for use in cattle, poul-try, and swine.

A healthier gut leads to a healthier animal, avoiding additional antibiotic treat-ment. The next time you hear about "antibiotics" being fed to meat animals, please dig a little deeper. You may find it's a product that helps animals digest feed better, which makes them more sustainable—and helps avoid having to treat them with antibiotics important to human medicine.

Birds are known for also having coccidia (a little protozoan) everywhere, so flocks are fed a coccidiostat to keep them healthy. One veterinarian told me, "If you don't control them, it leads to more antibiotic usage in birds. Coccidia can survive many types of cleaning and disinfecting."

Chickens are susceptible because they are so much younger; broilers (chickens for meat) are typically seven to eight weeks old when processed. Because of improved breeding practices, broilers grow very fast, which makes their immune, circulatory, and digestive systems very fast acting. Coccidiostats help reduce the risk of bad bacteria, which can lead to more diseases. Most chickens are given an ionophore or a nonantibiotic coccidiostat for an FDA-approved amount of time to prevent intestinal disease.

These are the antibiotics that comprise the majority being given to farm animals. As outlined, they aren't the antibiotics effective with humans, but they do help animals. The next time you hear about "animals filled with antibiotics," ask your-self if the drugs in question are important for human medicine or tools to improve the health of farm animals and your food safety.

A VETERINARIAN'S PERSPECTIVE ON ANTIBIOTICS

"We use as little as possible and as much as necessary," says veterinarian Dr. Leah Dorman. She and her husband are raising three teenaged girls on a farm in Ohio. Dorman was assistant state veterinarian for the Ohio Department of Agriculture.

She now works for an animal health company, but remains devoted to keep-ing poultry healthy. "For those of us passionate about animal health, the fact that antibiotics prevent suffering is key," she says. Leah believes "no antibiotics ever" and "antibiotic-free" has the potential to create animal care issues. "I had the opportunity to talk with a turkey grower who provides meat to Subway and he told me, 'The company wants antibiotic-free and they're willing to pay for it. But, that means when these turkeys get sick, I have to watch a percentage of them die.'"

"And from a sustainability standpoint, antibiotics help keep flocks healthy. Healthy birds utilize less feed, which means less land is needed, leading to a decreased carbon footprint."

She firmly believes antibiotic stewardship involves using as little as possible and as much as necessary.

> Withholding treatment for sick animals is unacceptable. Animals not treated could have internal issues that would cause issues during processing . . . We need to do what's right by the animal and for public health. There are multiple safeguards in place to assure the chicken we feed our families is safe, wholesome, and free of any unsafe residue. When meat is labeled 'antibiotic-free,' it simply means that the animal was raised without the benefit of antibiotics. I am concerned some animals are left to suffer when they get sick in situations where antibiotics have been taken away as a tool for ethical animal care.

> As a mother, farmer and vet, I love the fact that there are so many choices at the grocery store. If it makes you feel better to get antibiotic-free meat, then I think that's great. However, sometimes those choices have unintended consequences, and that's what worries me—the care of the animals.

> As veterinarians, we take an oath to protect animal health, promote human health, and prevent animal suffering. I wholeheartedly support consumer choice—I just want to ensure consumers have the chance to make informed choices. In my view, it's about finding a responsible balance.

RESPONSIBLE BALANCE

Responsible balance should not be about elimination, but about reviewing the science, checking the protocol, and being sure there is a system is in place to prevent overuse in *both* animals and humans. The FDA has repeatedly said one cannot draw definite conclusions from any direct comparisons between the quantity of antibiotics sold for use in humans and the quantity sold for use in animals.

The FDA's Veterinary Feed Directive (VFD) rule ensures the judicious use of medically important antimicrobials in food-producing animals. Starting in January 2017, the VFD required veterinarians to work with farmers and ranchers to make clinical judgments about animal health, have sufficient information about how the animal is managed, and provide for any necessary follow-up. This VFD means veterinarians will determine what can legally be used in feed or water for food-producing animals.[64]

If you worry about antibiotics in your meat, remember there is a system in place to protect you. There are no unsafe or harmful residues in your meat. If an antibiotic is used on the farm, federal rules require the antibiotic residues to have cleared the animals' systems before they can be slaughtered. For approved antibiotics, the FDA and USDA have extensive monitoring and testing programs to make sure your meat does not contain antibiotic residues.

The debate of antibiotic resistance is an important one—and more complex than a claim on a meat package. "When comparing humans and food-producing animals by body weight, humans consume 10 times more antibiotics per unit of body weight than farm animals."[65]

As you stand at the meat case, buy the kind of meat that will best power your family—regardless of label claims.

24. Is Meat Messing with Your Hormones?

PUMPING UP THE MEAT

When I was a teenager, I drew comic cows. These cows often had big muscles—biceps like Olympic athletes. I drew them because they were cute—and as a 5'5" female, I know how strong cattle can be. Never did I consider that someday people would think farm animals are "pumped up" on drugs.

> **Food Truth**
> Hormones are in everything.

I have since learned that apparently people think cows are on crazy amounts of steroids. That is *not* the case. It's also not the case with chickens, turkeys, or pigs.

Yes, your bacon, burger, chicken wings, turkey breast, and brats all have hormones. Hormones are in *all* food.

The big questions and food myths:

- *Is my meat pumped full of hormones?*
- *Are hormones only used to help a farmer make money?*
- *Aren't hormones making animals huge and hurting their health?*

WHAT ABOUT BIG BREASTS?

There is a myth that chickens and turkeys have big breasts because they're on hormones. Both chickens and turkeys are bred to grow larger breasts; it's in the genetics (breeding in response to consumer demand). The use of growth hormone has not been approved in raising chickens for 50 years. Same with turkeys. And pigs.

To be clear, no hormones are fed, injected, sprayed, sprinkled, or otherwise given to swine or poultry. No chickens, turkeys, pigs, or Cornish game hens have added hormones—regardless of the label claim. There aren't even any such products manufactured to give to them!

Historically, the USDA recognized the potential for consumer confusion with product labeling. For example, some companies began requesting approval to label chicken as "hormone free" (which is impossible, for those keeping track) and "no added hormones." The USDA started requiring these claims could not be used to market poultry unless the claim was followed by the disclaimer "Federal regulations prohibit the use of hormones in poultry."

Will you ingest hormones if you eat turkey or chicken? Yes. Will you ingest hormones if you eat kale? Yes. Does your bacon include hormones? Yes. Hormones are the chemical messengers of life—all living things have hormones.

So do you. Your body produces estrogen each day: 513,000 monograms if you're a woman who's not pregnant, only to be topped by 19,600,000 nanograms of estrogen produced daily by a pregnant woman. Men produce 136,000 nanograms of estrogen a day (and therefore should reserve comment about female hormones).[66]

BEEF AND HORMONES

What does this have to do with the discussion of hormones in meat? Plenty. Given the sensationalism around beef filled with hormones, perspective is important. Let's take a look at levels of steroids in an eight-ounce serving of common foods, listed in nanograms (which is one-billionth of a gram).[67]

Table 5

Eight-Ounce Serving	Nanograms of Steroids
Soy flour defatted	755,000,000
Tofu	113,500,000
Pinto beans	900,000
White bread	300,000
Peanuts	100,000
Eggs	555
Butter	310
Milk	32
Beef (implanted steer)	7
Beef (nonimplanted steer)	5

As you can see, there's plenty of food with higher levels of hormones than eight ounces of beef. Before we delve into why implants are used in some beef cattle and how it's done, let's take a look at human use of hormones.

Consider birth control pills, testosterone therapy, and hormone therapy. What hormone dosage are you ingesting? As an example, let's say a 170-pound woman on low-dose birth control takes about 0.48 milligrams of estrogen monthly (not to mention the progesterone) for 21 of 28 days every month. If she—or anyone else on hormone therapy—stops taking it, does the hormone stop working?

Yes, hormones stop working if you no longer take them. Hormones don't pile up in your system; they do not have a build-up effect that prevents pregnancy, causes cancer, or turns you into the Incredible Hulk. The same is true in both humans and beef cattle. Hormones don't build up; there is no residue in your meat.

Why are cattle implanted with hormones? Because male calves are castrated to prevent aggression, they lose their hormone-producing organ providing small amounts of these or similar hormones to allow them to regain some of the growth rate they would naturally have as bulls. Implants, like human hormones, are actually naturally produced hormones.

The amounts of hormones in an implant are a fraction of the natural production of mature bulls or heifers. A 1,300-pound steer is implanted with 30 mg of estrogen to last 150 days. And that's all the hormones he gets. Compare this to the ingested hormones of the woman on birth control.

Again, as a mom of a daughter, I understand why hormones freak parents out. They sound scary, but hormones serve a natural purpose in all living things. Implants have been used in beef cattle since 1954 because they help reduce the carbon footprint of meat. Cattle with implants can convert their feed to muscle more efficiently and grow 15 percent faster during the finishing phase, which is when cattle are being prepared to provide the highest-quality meat. More feed efficiency and faster growth means less environmental impact.

How are these implants put in cattle? Implants are about the size of an Advil tablet and put under the skin on the backside of the ear. The implant is put there because the ear never enters the meat supply; the steer never has hormones shot in them. Research from Iowa shows that hormone implants have no effect on beef quality or safety.[68]

When you stand at the meat case and worry about hormones, consider this: the USDA and all of the major countries' scientific bodies, including the European Union, the Academy of Nutrition and Dietetics, and the Journal of Clinical Nutrition, have all said beef from natural and organic programs is not safer, more nutritious, more wholesome, or different in appearance compared with beef from animals that have received implants.

WHY EAT MEAT?

What matters most is that your family has high-quality protein. The 2015–2020 *Dietary Guidelines* say the recommendation for the meats, poultry, and eggs subgroup at the 2,000-calorie level is 26 ounce-equivalents per week.

Why? There are many reasons meat matters. The *Dietary Guidelines* show meat is an important source of nutrients in addition to protein, including B vitamins (e.g., niacin, vitamin B_{12}, vitamin B_6, and riboflavin), selenium, choline, phosphorus, zinc, copper, vitamin D, and vitamin E).

Nutrients provided by various types of protein foods differ. For example, meats provide the most zinc, and poultry provides the most niacin. Red meats, poultry, and seafood provide heme iron, which is more bioavailable than the nonheme iron found in plant sources, and this is especially important for young children and pregnant women and those capable of becoming pregnant.

The bottom line of the meat case is this: worrying about nutrition for your body is more important than fussing over hormones that are tested, highly regulated, and have been safely used for more than 60 years. But records show women, especially girls ages 14 to 18, are not getting enough protein.[69]

What happens when a body doesn't have enough protein? The human body cannot function normally and may experience muscle loss (unexpected weight loss), fatigue, low sex drive, depression, anxiety, and anemia.

Up to 25 percent of girls in the United States are iron deficient—not anemic, but do not consume enough iron, according to a 1996 study on cognitive functioning. When the girls were supplemented with iron, both their verbal learning and memory improved. Eating meat is an excellent way to improve iron levels in girls—as well address the other side effects of protein deprivation.[70] Protein is also shown to help prevent muscle loss with aging, improve metabolic functioning, and manage weight to avoid obesity and type 2 diabetes.[71]

Remember, when it comes to chicken, pork, and turkey, there are never any hormones injected, sprayed, or fed to the animals. Most beef is from implanted cattle because it is more sustainable.

You choose the protein that is right for your family; I choose meat that meets my cooking needs, looks good, and is priced right—regardless of hormone label claims.

25. The Mass Production of Education, Medication, and Food

THE SIZE OF HOSPITALS, SCHOOLS . . . AND FARMS

"I guess that's just the way it is today," another mom said about the farm she visited. "It's just mass production." She wasn't upset, just making an observation.

We had been discussing family medical situations, so I asked, "How does your family choose hospitals?"

"We typically go to a large system with the best specialists."

Her kids go to a school where they will have over 600 students in their graduating class. In a new building, filled with technology, and measured by the latest standards. Mine goes to a small school

> **Food Truth**
> Housing is used to protect animals—and your food—from nature.

where all the teachers know their name and they have different opportunities because it is a smaller system.

When I mentioned how that was the same as agriculture, I saw a light go on. Larger farms specialize in their product—and face more regulations than small operations—similar to large hospitals with specialists. Larger farms often utilize more technology, have newer facilities, and have very clear standards—like large schools. It's not that larger is better; it's just a sign of our times. Likewise, small is not wrong—it's a different experience.

There is no need to feel guilty because of the size of farm you are supporting—nor should you buy foods because a label makes a claim about farm size. Community-supported agriculture (CSA), 5,000-acre farms, farmers' market vendors, and ranches with 5,000 head of cattle can all be good operators.

Good farms are good farms regardless of size—just like schools and hospitals.

The big questions and food myths:

- *Why are animals kept inside and not in nature?*
- *What are farmers hiding inside of those long metal buildings?*
- *Isn't it cruel to have animals so crowded?*

ANIMAL PILES

What do your dogs do during a storm or when they are seeking comfort? Crawl into your bed? Hover at your feet? Lie on top of each other? Crowding together is an animal's natural way of comforting themselves—whether keeping cool, staying warm, trying to get away from pesky flies, or getting out of the wind.

Farm animals are herders; it is their natural instinct to protect themselves. You may see that in a dirt feedlot where you see cattle "crowded" in a corner, or a chicken house where broilers gather together, but that is their natural behavior.

THE JOY OF GROWING CHICKENS

Aaron believes it is a privilege to farm with his family on their Hartly, Delaware farm. He is the fourth generation on a farm started in 1911. Their family raises 550,000 roaster chickens annually in three chicken houses for one of the major poultry brands.

Does 550,000 chickens a year seem like "big ag" to you? I asked Aaron why they have so many chickens—and you may be surprised that this is still very much a family farm.

"Our chicken operation may seem large to most but we raise that many to provide for three families within the Thompson family. The manure is also a perk because we use it on our corn and wheat crops." Poultry manure is particularly good fertilizer because of its nitrogen and urea content.

In addition to the roaster chickens, Aaron's family farms 1,200 acres of corn, soybeans, and soft red winter wheat. "Our soybeans and corn stay on the Delmarva peninsula to feed the poultry. The wheat is milled in Pennsylvania for cookies or pretzels."

Contrary to what you may believe, no chickens raised for meat are in cages. None. Regardless of whether the label claims "cage free" or not, broiler chickens are not in cages. Because their lifespan is usually less than two months, they do not reach sexual maturity and become aggressive toward each other. Any "cage-free" claim on chicken meat is another marketing mistruth.

Because Aaron is with the chickens every day, I asked him to explain how the chickens are housed.

"The chickens are housed in a cage-free building where they are free to roam. Antibiotic-free and hormone-free feed, along with fresh water, are available to them at all times through an automatic computer-controlled system. The computer controller also keeps the birds comfortable by either heating or cooling their building."

Like laying hens, hogs, and turkeys, broilers are placed inside the buildings to control their environment while limiting their exposure to outside bacteria, predators, and diseases.

Biosecurity—keeping chickens safe from diseases—is a pretty big deal in the chicken world. I think poultry farms have more protocol than some hospitals.

"All equipment that enters the poultry house must be cleaned and sanitized before entering. Dedicated footwear to be worn at the poultry facilities is worn and also dipped into a footbath with sanitizer before entering. All of the drinking water is treated with chlorine, much like municipal water. Copper sulfate and vitamins are injected at specific times in the drinking water to maintain a healthy bird," said Aaron.

CLOSED BARNS KEEP ANIMALS HEALTHY

The same is true for turkeys. They are raised in scientifically designed barns, not cages. Since avian influenza destroyed 50 million turkeys and egg-laying hens in 2015, biosecurity is especially important across all poultry farms. Although the cause is still being investigated, there is reason to believe that migrating birds are responsible for the devastating influenza.

Hogs also require tight biosecurity in their environmentally controlled barns, after more than 7 million piglets were killed by porcine epidemic diarrhea virus in 2014. This virus most likely arrived from China and was unlike anything the pork business had seen.[72]

Do animals live behind closed doors? Yes, the doors are closed and barns are closely monitored to keep animals healthy. Is this because of overcrowding confined operations, big ag, or factory farms? No. Animals like to herd together, and if you're a visitor, you'll likely see this behavior because they don't know you. Nature is cruel, but farmers and ranchers build barns to try to protect animals from nature. Farm animals are healthier and more comfortable than when they were in the mud 50 years ago. Also important to remember: animals don't grow or produce when they are not in healthy conditions. Big isn't bad, small isn't bad— they're just different.

26. Does Your Burger Damage the Environment?

COW BURPS AND THE BIG PICTURE

One of the concerns about meat, particularly beef, comes by way of methane. If you're not aware, a 1,500-pound cow can out-burp and pass gas more than your crazy college roommate, but that doesn't make them industrial greenhouse gas producers. Generation of the electricity that powers your house created 12 times more greenhouse gas emissions than the methane of *all* the livestock in the United States, according to the EPA in 2014. Transportation in the United

> **Food Truth**
>
> Sustainability is complex and essential to family businesses.

States makes nearly nine times more greenhouse gas emissions than methane from livestock.[73]

After working in developing countries and seeing the consequence of lower environmental standards in countries such as Egypt, the former Soviet states, and South Africa, I believe sustainability is a global issue. We wring our hands over fairly minor issues in the United States, while doing little to learn about or offer solutions in other parts of the world.

Sustainability also involves a local component, as the well-being of local family businesses includes an economic component. True sustainability supports the environment and allows for the growth of family businesses like farms. A sustainable business is one that is passed from generation to generation. Ultimately, sustainability is about survival. Survival of the environment, resilience of a business, and the opportunity for both to thrive.

The big questions and food myths:

- *Is it environmentally irresponsible to eat meat?*
- *Is grass-fed more sustainable and corn bad for cattle?*
- *Why is sustainability more than just the environment?*

IS CORN-FED OR GRASS-FED THE MOST RESPONSIBLE?

Corn-fed or grass-fed seems to be one of the big questions in the meat case. Somewhere the myth came into play that cattle shouldn't eat corn and grass is better. First, from a sustainability standpoint grass-fed beef is not better for the environment. According to Dr. Jude Capper in a Washington State study, cattle fed grain use 76 percent less water and 49 percent less feed on 45 percent less land. The output is equally as impressive; cattle on grain make 51 percent less manure and 42 percent less carbon.[74]

In other words, if cattle stayed on grass pastures instead of being fed corn for four to five months at a feed yard, there would be more land required—and the cattle would be producing more greenhouse grass emission. Corn-fed is defined as cattle that are fed corn to finish out their meat. This is not done for the farmer's profitability, but to enhance the flavor of the beef.

If you choose grass-fed because you prefer the taste, great. Just know that it's not a more responsible way to produce meat—nor is corn bad for cattle. Cattle eating corn digest it in such a way that it adds marbling to the meat, providing an impression of tenderness and flavor. Contrary to popular claims, corn has provided energy for livestock for centuries.

Cattle love corn; they are not being force-fed something they do not enjoy. My daughter actually conducted her third-grade science fair experiment on whether cows preferred corn or hay (the green stuff usually made of grass, alfalfa, etc.). Corn won every time. In fact, it wasn't uncommon for cows to tip their feed tub upside down looking for more corn before they even thought about the hay. Both types of feed are necessary to keep cattle healthy—just as your body requires the right balance of a variety of food.

"It's not natural for cattle to digest corn" is the claim some make. We adjust cow diets gradually to give time for the gut bacteria to adapt. Just as in humans, infants shouldn't be started on whole milk before developing the right gut bacteria, which happens around one year of age. If those bacteria aren't developed, the toddler may need more time rather than just being labeled lactose intolerant. The same is true in corn; we slowly increase corn in the diet.

My breakfast often includes a high dose of protein like Greek yogurt or peanut butter or eggs because I'm like many women and struggle to get enough protein. However, I rarely have a problem with cramming in carbohydrates. When coaching cross-country, I need carbs for ongoing energy, but my body stores up energy like a hibernating bear if I continue the same carb consumption when not as active. Cattle also need a combination of protein and carbs; their nutrition is scientifically balanced on a weekly basis, so they are getting more attention than a human diet.

Corn isn't bad. Grass isn't bad. Both are necessary at different times in an animal's life cycle, whether beef or dairy. Beef cattle spend the vast majority of their life on grass. When it comes time for a beef animal to finish growing for a steak or burger with flavor, those animals most often go to a feedlot (an operation that specializes in growing beef for meat).

Keep in mind that 85 percent of grazing lands in the United States is unsuitable for growing crops, so don't have angst that your choice to eat meat is causing land to be wasted. The same is true in Canada; much of their 11 million hectares of rangeland are amenable to pasture but can't be cropped.[75]

Dr. Jude Capper has done extensive research on livestock's environmental impact at Washington State and Cornell Universities. In a recent *Wall Street Journal* article, Jude talks about improvements in animal agriculture that have led to a reduced environmental impact of eating meat.[76]

> Feedlot cattle spend 70 percent to 80 percent of their lives on pasture, and only the last four or five months in a feedlot, where they eat grains, legumes, forage, and byproducts from human feed and fiber production. The healthy, well-cared-for cattle I have seen in feedlots from the U.S. and Europe to Australia and South Africa don't fit the "factory farm" label. A feedlot is not utopia, but neither is a grass pasture in the midst of a six-month drought.
>
> American beef producers have continually improved how they breed, feed, and care for cattle while maintaining the high safety, quality, and taste standards for which U.S. beef is renowned. In 2007, each pound of beef produced required 19 percent less feed, 33 percent less land, 12 percent less water, and 9 percent less fossil fuels than equivalent production in 1977, and was associated with 19 percent less manure and a 16 percent decrease in the carbon footprint. That's from a peer-reviewed study I published in 2011 largely based on data from the U.S. Department of Agriculture. These are huge achievements for an industry often incorrectly described as an environmental villain.
>
> If feedlot critics would have us return cattle production to pastures alone, they are not considering the environmental impact. Based on my peer-reviewed, published research, to keep producing 26 billion pounds of U.S. beef each year from grass-fed systems would require 135 million additional acres of land, 468 billion more gallons of water, and an increase in carbon emissions equivalent to adding 27 million cars to the road.
>
> Put simply, feedlot beef is not a waste of water. Cereal crops use less water per pound, but they don't provide the same range of nutrients as beef, nor can they be produced on low-quality pasture and rangeland. Claims, meanwhile, that 70 percent of U.S. corn production goes to feeding livestock are wildly inaccurate, as are estimates based on that figure of how much water is used in raising feedlot cattle. Only 9 percent of total U.S. corn production in 2014 was grown for beef cattle feed.
>
> Beef producers do everything they can to preserve the land, water and air on which they rely. The EPA regulates potential pollution through nutrient management plans, permits, and annual reporting. More than 60 percent of beef feedlots regularly test groundwater for environmental quality; 75 percent test the nutrient content of cattle manure; and 93 percent test soil nutrient levels to make sure they don't over-apply manure onto cropland. Unfortunately, ammonia is emitted from the breakdown of nitrogen in manure from all animals, farmed or wild, but nitrogen in cattle feed is being reduced.

Jude believes we should eat safe, affordable, high-quality food that minimizes negative impacts on the environment: "Feedlot beef is my choice for my family."

SUSTAINABILITY ACROSS THE MEAT CASE

Work has been done to improve sustainability across the meat case, from beef to pork to turkeys. Wanda, the Minnesota pork farmer, talked about their focus.

"The technology is there to help us be more sustainable. Our hogs use less water and less food. Manure is recycled from under the barn and it's a far better nutrient. It's the ultimate recycling program."

Sietsema Farms in western Michigan, where three generations farm side by side and have reduced feed resources more than 20 percent in the last 20 years, have turned to poop for power. The Sietsemas recently built a biomass system that converts turkey litter into energy that powers their grain elevator, where grain is stored and processed into feed. It's a clean waste disposal system with a zero-carbon footprint generating the energy equivalent of nearly 8,500 barrels of oil annually. That's enough to provide electricity for up to 400 average American homes. The system not only sustains the environment, it sustains the family farm and their employees. As long as turkeys are still raised there, the energy source won't run out.

"We want to be able to have a successful farm that will continue into the next generations," says Harley Sietsema. "We want to preserve the environment and be a blessing to the communities that we reside in."[77]

As you stand at the meat case, you have every right to choose the environmental standard for your family, but please know there is a decreasing carbon footprint from animal agriculture. This trend will continue as long as livestock producers are allowed to increase their efficiency.

27. There Is No Singular "Right" Way to Buy or Grow Food

WE ARE DIFFERENT, WE ARE ONE

As reported by a number of news sources in February 2016, Justice Ruth Bader Ginsburg was the U.S. Supreme Court's most liberal member at that time, whereas Justice Antonin Scalia was its most conservative. Yet they treasured one another. Ginsburg's tribute to Scalia at his passing started with "We are different, we are one, different in our interpretation of written texts, one in our reverence for the Constitution and the institution we serve."

> **Food Truth**
>
> Organic farming is about production methods, not nutritional value.

If two opinionated Supreme Court judges with opposite opinions can respect each other, shouldn't we all be making that effort? The lack of civil discourse in our society erodes the chance to have a real conversation about issues that matter. For example, the way food is grown. Is it really possible a label on food is more important than civility? I think not. Is it likely marketing on healthy foods is just as challenging as marketing on junk food? Decide for yourself, but after 15 years of researching the topic, I'd say absolutely.

The big questions and food myths:

- *Is organic meat better for my family?*
- *Are there fewer hormones and antibiotics in organic?*
- *Is organic more environmentally friendly?*

WHEN IS A STEAK A STEAK?

There is no singular right way to raise meat. A label should not infer superiority or inferiority. A brand making those marketing claims on food labels is best avoided, in my opinion. Marketing on labels is confusing and leads to guilt.

Meat case packages making the "natural" claim were 38 percent in 2015, up 16 percent from 2004, according to *Dynamics of the Meat Case* from the 2016 Annual Meat Conference.[78] Is our beef 16 percent more natural? Likely not. Is our bias as grocery store shoppers buying the "natural" label that much higher? Apparently so, or meat marketers would not be adding that label to the package.

As far as organic product claims, beef and chicken both made significantly more claims. According to the same presentation, chicken was up nearly 5 percent in 2015 as compared to 2007.

"What am I supposed to be looking for in my meat? Isn't organic always better?" asked a female CEO in healthcare, after one of my speaking programs.

"You decide what is the right meat for you based upon your family's needs and priorities. Not on brand, label claims, guilt, or status symbol," was my quick response. We talked more about the complexities of making that decision; the fact that organic is a production style overseen by the marketing branch of the USDA, not a nutritional guarantee, and that there are sustainability complications that many don't take into consideration (e.g. more meat wasted, greater land use, less efficient feed use).

Janeal Yancey, a PhD meat scientist at the University of Arkansas, explained the differences between three meat labels on her blog *Mom at the Meat Counter.*

> I am not trying to say that meat labeled as 'Natural' or 'Organic' or 'Grass-fed' is any better or worse than any other meat you may find in a grocery store or a restaurant. I will tell you that it is also not any safer or more nutritious than other meat. I just tell people, eat what you like, and when it comes to food labels, know what you are paying for.

> 1. **Organic**: Animals must be only fed organic feed and allowed to graze only organically managed pastures. They are not to be given hormones or any other growth-promoting agents, and only allowed to be given vaccines when they are not sick (nothing else). There are requirements that they must be allowed access to outdoors. All of these regulations are certified by agencies accredited through [the] USDA. In order to place the USDA organic seal on the label of a product, it must be made with 95 percent or greater organic ingredients. Meat labeled as "organic" is expensive because it costs a lot to produce.

2. **Natural:** Lots of people think that "Natural" is the same as "Organic." It is not. According to [the] USDA Food Safety and Inspection Service, a product with the word "Natural" on the label must be "a product containing no artificial ingredient or added color and is only minimally processed. Minimal processing means that the product was processed in a manner that does not fundamentally alter the product. The label must include a statement explaining the meaning of the term natural (such as 'no artificial ingredients; minimally processed')."

3. **Grass-fed:** Producers feed cattle grain for the last three or four months of their life, an efficient way to get the cattle to gain weight and fatten to a point where American consumers like to eat beef. Most of us like juicy, tender beef, and that comes from marbled beef. Grass-fed beef is generally leaner and has a stronger flavor than grain-fed beef. To be labeled "grass (forage) fed" meat (most likely beef or lamb), the animal must have only been allowed to eat grass or hay for its entire life (except milk when they are babies). Grass feeding takes a longer time to get cattle large enough to slaughter, and there is not as much meat on grass-fed beef. So, it costs more.

There are many claims on meat packages from marketing claims to certifications to confusing nutrition information. The USDA Agricultural Marketing Service manages the "Certified Organic" seal to ensure food is grown to guidelines addressing, among many factors, soil quality, animal raising practices, pest and weed control, and use of additives. Organic meat regulations require that animals are raised in living conditions accommodating their natural behaviors (like the ability to graze on pasture—though no stipulation is made about what percentage of their life is outside), fed 100 percent organic feed and forage, and not administered antibiotics or hormones.

As described in the dairy section, the most significant difference between organic and conventional beef is the use of antibiotics and hormones. You decide what the right meat for your family is; just know organic is not about nutrition, but a production style.

The USDA's Food Safety Inspection Service shares their "Animal Production Claims Outline of Current Process." They list unapprovable claims—those they won't approve for meat—as the following: antibiotic free, hormone free, residue free, residue tested, naturally raised naturally grown, drug free, chemical free, organic, organically raised.[79] How many of these have added confusion to you meat-buying confusion in the past?

If you wish to evaluate the nutrition of your meat—or any other food in the grocery store—look to the Nutrition Facts Panel on your food. The Nutrition Facts Panel is the best place to get your information, or seek out expert advice from a science-based registered dietitian, who may be available at your grocery store.

Personally, I choose conventionally raised meat with as few marketing claims as possible. Science supports this choice, and I find conventionally raised to be the most responsible for animal welfare, as well as more sustainable—considering the waste that occurs with organic meat.

28. Are You Growing Bacteria?

HAND HYGIENE IS NEEDED, EVEN IN HOSPITALS

We live in a society where only 5 percent of people who use the bathroom wash their hands enough to kill germs that can cause illness. Thirty-three percent of hand washers didn't use soap, and 10 percent skipped washing in a recent study. According to the U.S. Centers for Disease Control (CDC), people need to vigorously wash their hands for 15 to 20 seconds to kill any dangerous bacteria. Most of us wash for six seconds.[80]

> **Food Truth**
>
> Food safety starts on the farm and ends in your kitchen.

Unfortunately, hand washing is even a problem in hospitals; health experts say poor hand cleanliness is a factor in infections that kills tens of thousands each year—infections that are acquired at the hospital. The CDC estimates that 1 of every 20 patients in the United States gets a hospital-acquired infection each year. "We've known for over 150 years that good hand hygiene prevents patients from getting infections," said Dr. John Jernigan, an epidemiologist at the CDC. "However, it's been a very chronic and difficult problem to [get] adherence levels up as high as we'd like them to be."[81]

Isn't it ironic that we are so concerned about what's in our food but we don't take time to wash our hands? Hands that are laden with bacteria, especially after a person uses the restroom and doesn't wash with soap.

Jernigan said, "For a healthcare worker, keeping their hands clean is the single most important thing they can do to protect their patients."

The same is true in your kitchen. The single most important thing you can do is wash your hands properly. Before you worry about what's on your meat, worry about what's on you! The second most important thing is washing the utensils and surfaces that come into contact with raw meat. Finally, the third most important factor is to cook your meat properly.

The big questions and food myths:

- *Is my food safer today?*
- *Where do most food safety violations happen?*

BACTERIA: GOOD OR BAD?

Even if your kitchen looks spotless, it likely has more bacteria than any other location in your house. Dishrags, the handle to your kitchen faucet, cutting boards, and surfaces where you place raw meat are breeding grounds for bacteria if not properly cleaned.

Bacteria happen. We don't live in a perfectly sanitary world.

Why are there bacteria in meat? Does that mean it's dirty? Janeal Yancey, the Meat Counter Mom from the University of Arkansas, said the United States has one of the safest food supplies in the world.

"We're doing a better job of controlling pathogens than we ever have. There is bacteria on everything. They live everywhere . . . we're finding there are lots of good bacteria that live in our body. They live in and on animals, as well. There are also bacteria that cause disease. Some of them, it only takes one to two organisms, maybe 10, that can make you ill."

That does not mean you should avoid meat. It is an important part of getting protein, iron, B_{12}, and other nutrients. Keeping those nasty organisms at bay is pretty simple—cook meat to the recommended temperature and clean up focused on bacteria.

The USDA Food Safety Information Service recommends four steps to safely prepare and serve food.

1. *Clean:* Wash your hands with warm water and soap for 20 seconds and sanitize surfaces, utensils, and cutting boards with one tablespoon of bleach in one gallon of water.
2. *Separate:* Do not cross-contaminate. Keep raw meat, poultry, fish, and their juices away from other food. After cutting raw meats, wash cutting board, utensils, and countertops with hot, soapy water.
3. *Cook:* Use a food thermometer to ensure it's cooked to the right temperature.
   - All raw beef, pork, lamb and veal steaks, chops, and roasts should be cooked to a minimum internal temperature of 145°F.
   - Ground beef, pork, lamb, and veal needs to be cooked to 160°F.
   - All poultry needs an internal temperature of 165°F.
4. *Chill:* Refrigerate promptly. Perishable food should not be left out more than two hours at room temperature—one hour when the temperature is above 90°F.

In order to have the best meat, the USDA recommends to cook or freeze fresh poultry, fish, ground meats, and variety meats within two days; other beef, veal, lamb, or pork should be cooked or frozen within three to five days.

MAGIC IN A MEAT THERMOMETER

What is greatest food safety concern regarding meat?

"Ground beef and ground meats because consumers still want to determine how they've cooked their meat with their eyes and by meat color. People need to use a meat thermometer. Sometimes it browns early, sometimes it browns late. If a burger or ground meat isn't cooked properly, it can result in sickness or a poor meat eating experience. You cannot eat a rare hamburger and expect to be safe from Salmonella, E. coli, or Listeria," said Janeal.

Is there something wrong with the way our meats are processed?

"No, meat is processed more safely today than ever. The meat in the middle of a whole muscle will stay relatively sanitary because it remains untouched by knives or humans. However, with a burger, bacteria from the environmentally exposed surface are ground up. The center needs to cook to 160°F to kill the bacteria. Looking at the color is NOT a good indicator. For example, when grilling burgers, they can cook on the outside, killing the bacteria there. However, the bacteria can still be alive on the inside. A meat thermometer will protect you from that," Janeal explained.

A common question is if animals are dirty because they live in manure. How can you tell if bacteria are growing on your meat?

"You can't tell if there are pathogenic bacteria. But if meat has been stored at improper temperatures (like when you took too long to get home from the grocery store,), throw it out. "Smell it. If it stinks, you're smelling spoilage organism—throw it out," urged Janeal.

MEAT SAFETY CONTROL POINTS

People may break safety rules when thawing out frozen meat, usually because they are in a hurry. Note these thawing pointers from the USDA:

- Thawing in the refrigerator: The refrigerator allows slow, safe thawing. Don't let meat and poultry juices drip onto other food.
- Thawing in cold water: Place food in a leak-proof plastic bag for faster thawing. Submerge in cold tap water. Change the water every 30 minutes. Cook immediately after thawing.
- Thawing in the microwave: Cook meat and poultry immediately after microwave thawing.

There are more checkpoints and tests to keep your meat safe today than at any point in history. The key is following the right food safety steps in your kitchen.

Table 6   Meat Case Food Truths

Food Myth	Food Truth
Animals are abused to produce meat.	**Food Truth 3: Animal welfare is an hourly concern on farms and ranches.** It is not an oxymoron to raise animals for food and treat them with respect.
Farm animal antibiotic use is responsible for humans developing antibiotic resistance.	**Food Truth 2: Antibiotics have benefits.** Residues aren't present, and 87 percent of antibiotics used in farm animals are not used in humans.
Meat is pumped full of hormones.	**Food Truth 1: Hormones are in everything.** Hormones are the chemical messengers of life. They are in every product, including plant-based foods.
Cattle in feedlots, pigs in pens, and poultry not roaming the range are wrong.	**Food Truth 4: Housing is used to protect animals— and your food—from nature.** A balanced diet and clean bedding, along with protecting animals from each other and the elements, make for safe food.
Eating meat hurts the environment.	**Food Truth 12: Sustainability is complex and essential to family businesses.** Environmental audits, technology, and family business survival skills all make up a truly sustainable model.
Organic is always the most nutritious and ethical choice.	**Food Truth 5: Organic farming is about production methods, not nutritional value.** Meat, organic or not, is a nutritious and necessary part of your diet—regardless of how it was produced.
Today's farming methods make my meat unsafe.	**Food Truth 11: Food safety starts on the farm and ends in your kitchen.** Proper cleaning, keeping bacteria off your cutting surfaces, and cooking meat thoroughly go a long way in protecting your family.

Part VI: Bread and Baking Aisle

The amber waves of grain have turned into an ambiguous guilt trip. How do you know if gluten is good, why sugar is demonized, and how to not be overwhelmed by baking if you're not Betty Crocker? This section will help you unravel the mystery of bread and baked goods.

"*If you desire peace, cultivate justice, but at the same time cultivate the fields to produce more bread; otherwise there will be no peace.*"

—Nobel Laureate Norman Borlaug

29. Saving Our Soil

HEALTHY SOIL GROWS HEALTHY PLANTS FOR BETTER BAKING

Do you know what stores 10 percent of the world's carbon dioxide? Soil. Soil is a carbon sink that stores more carbon dioxide than the terrestrial vegetation and the atmosphere combined. When soil is disturbed, carbon dioxide is released into the environment and contributes to global warming.

Soil is the foundation of food. It is the key to great baking. Are you thinking you don't want dirt in your kitchen? Soil isn't dirt—it's essential to healthy plants that make up flour, sugar, corn meal, etc.

Sadly, an area about the size of Costa Rica of topsoil is lost each year. It can take more than 500 years to form two centimeters of topsoil, which is the good stuff that crops grow in. Nearly 50,000 square kilometers of topsoil is lost each year due to water and wind erosion.[82]

That's a huge loss—one that farmers take very seriously as they grow food for your baking aisle.

The big questions and food myths:

- *Isn't soil suffering with today's farming practices?*
- *Don't farmers just pour chemicals on the soil?*

HEALTHY PLANTS COME FROM SOIL THAT'S ALIVE!

The Mississippi River carves out beautiful green hills and woodlands in western Wisconsin. East of LaCross, a pretty historic town a couple of hours southeast of Minneapolis, is where Kevin Hoyer farms around 500 acres of soybeans, corn, and pasture with his wife, Jody.

Healthy water matters to the Hoyers; their farm has a trout stream on it, so they want to be sure the water can continue to support that. They use buffer strips (portions of land not planted with a crop) to provide more space between their field and the stream. Kevin said they have changed practices from the past as they have learned what hurts the environment as agronomy continues to advance; they are getting rid of insecticides and limiting things that can leach into water.

"We take conservation seriously," Kevin says. "We live and work in this environment, so we want to take care of it." He is also a certified crop advisor, meaning he advises other farmers on the science of soil and the nutrition of plants. You could call him a soil doctor.

As we talked after I spoke at a conference, Kevin emphasized plants need nutrition to survive—just like we do. Water and soil are a significant part of that equation. He believes his soil is more alive now due to updated practices.

Soil health has improved on Kevin's farm because he's changed how he works with the land—known as tillage practices. He uses no-till and minimal till to return soil tilth—the physical condition of soil (measured by soil particles, moisture content, aeration, drainage, etc.). No-till has become a common practice for many row crop farmers. No till (or minimal till) just means the land is not plowed, disked, or disturbed prior to planting to increase organic matter.

Kevin, like most farmers, judges soil nutrition based upon results from soil testing (from a probe that pulls up a soil sample in different parts of the field). He also has started planting cover crops to reduce erosion and help with nutrients in the soil. He points to less need for insecticides due to genetically modified seeds and integrated pest management as reasons for the improvement in soil health.

TECHNOLOGY PRESCRIBING SOIL SOLUTIONS

"The explosion of technology over the last decade has overshadowed the basics of agronomy," Kevin said, then explaining how farmers use fewer inputs (pesticides and fertilizers) because they can identify exactly where stresses are and then pinpoint what is needed and exactly where it is needed.

"GPS driven maps of fields, along with soil samples from different parts of the field (grid) and tissue samples (from the bean or corn plant) identify where specific nutrients are needed in that particular field. Equipment that allows fertilizer to be applied at a variable rate, meaning different parts of the field can get different amounts of product needed by the plants and/or soil. The equipment drives itself—tractors and sprayers are hands-free using the GPS map to drive, which keeps overlap to a minimum. Farmers produce as much product with as minimal negative environmental impacts," Kevin says, as he talks about how he plans crop rotation field by field before planting. "Plants also need protection to produce as much as they can."

Soil tests, past yields, and seed selections help him plan—along with how weedy the field is likely to be—soil moisture and what products are needed to grow the strongest plant. Micronutrients (e.g., nitrogen, calcium, etc.) are applied at a prescriptive rate according to what this information tells him just before planting. About the same time, a field is treated with an herbicide to kill weeds (this is called a pre-emergent since it's before the crop has emerged from the ground) at a rate approved by EPA. "Using a mix of herbicides at different timings provides multiple modes of action to reduce weed resistance. I apply residual herbicides (weed control that is active for four weeks) at a reduced rate, but it is important to keep other weeds from germinating," he said.

People often ask why farmers use weed control. Consider weeds in your flowerbed. Do they grow quickly? Can they choke out the good plants? The same is true in a field, though farmers actually apply herbicides and fertilizers at lower rates than homeowners because of concerns for the environment, the cost of the products, and the actual training/licensure to apply the products.

30,000 WEEDS, 3,000 NEMATODES, AND 10,000 INSECTS

Fields would be taken over by weeds and bugs if they were not sprayed. Why? This is what crop plants compete with in a field: 30,000 species of weeds, 3,000 species of nematodes, and 10,000 species of plant-eating insects.[83]

Kevin indicates the combination of residual and contact herbicide is the most effective and cost efficient for him to manage competition from weeds. The contact weed killer protects groundwater because they are applied at a lower rate. The contact herbicide—a product such as Round-Up you may use in your yard—is necessary to kill weeds that do grow and can damage the crop.

When the soil temperature is right and the fields aren't too wet, soybeans are then drilled in or corn is planted, both at very precise depths in the soil. Farmers are careful to monitor conditions during planting because a wet field can result in compacted soil, and cold ground means seeds don't germinate.

Once the plants are up, Kevin watches them for "hunger deficiencies." "The plants will tell you what they need. Is the plant showing symptoms of phosphorous, nitrogen, potassium, or other nutrient deficiency?" If so, he confirms his finding with a tissue test (sending a small piece of plant off to the lab) and then treats accordingly. It's kind of if your pet is showing a deficiency and then it gets the right nutrients.

The crop receives another dose of nitrogen when the plants are ankle high— nitrogen is a critical nutrient in plant growth. However, it can move with rain, so Kevin uses a nitrogen modeling program to determine the right amount, waiting for the right weather.

What is glyophosate and why do we need to know about it in the bakery aisle?

"Glyphosate is the active ingredient in Round-Up. It's applied after the soybeans are emerged to control weeds already growing," Kevin explained. To put this chemical into perspective: on an entire acre 32 ounces or less are sprayed a minimum of three months before harvest, the equivalent to a quart of milk sprayed across a football field.

The fields are then watched for insects and diseases. Kevin said some of the diseases just have to run their course in the plants, kind of like we have to let flu run its course. He selects all of his soybeans based upon disease tolerance so he doesn't have to apply fungicides to reduce the dependence on them.

He chooses to grow both GMO and non-GMO soybeans. He grows non-GMO for a premium in the export market. Kevin indicates the non-GMO soybeans typically cost $80 more an acre to grow and have lower yield.

Why grow GMO crops? Doesn't that mean more chemicals?

"The GMO soybeans grown in this country use less pesticides than non-GMO. The GMO trait is less invasive on beneficial insects or organisms, along with reducing chemical use," Kevin said.

When harvest is done, the soil doctor goes back into action. Kevin determines which field has more weed pressure and then will plant cover crop to keep soil in place and trap nutrients. And then the cycle begins all over again with planning for the following year.

Growing food like soybeans is an evolving process. Soil is a critical part of growing food for your baking—and farmers are using all the tools they have to be sure their soil is as healthy as possible.

30. Would You Like a Loaf of Guilt with Your Bread?

GLUTEN AS THE FOOD FAD DU JOUR

One of my friend's 15-year-old daughters recently spent over 30 minutes trying to find hard-shelled tacos. You know the kind—the yellow corn shells standard in the Mexican food section? She found them, but it was the label that took forever; she wanted taco shells without a gluten-free label. In the infamous words of a teenager: "Because it's stupid they put that on the label, it's just corn shells."

> **Food Truth**
> Grains are an important part of your diet.

A teenager clearly had a better grasp on gluten than most adults. *Merriam-Webster* defines gluten as a tenacious elastic protein substance especially of wheat flour that gives cohesiveness to dough. Other definitions say gluten is a substance present in cereal grains, especially wheat, that is responsible for the elastic texture of dough.

Milk, vegetables, and water have recently been labeled gluten-free. Why? If gluten was truly understood, would it need to be labeled? No. Gluten is undoubtedly the food fad du jour.

For an estimated 1 in every 100 people, celiac disease is a real concern. Celiac is a genetic autoimmune disorder, whereby eating gluten (a protein found in wheat, rye, and barley) triggers a digestive response that attacks the small intestine. Avoiding gluten is vital for their health.

But for the vast majority of people, grains are good in the diet. Grains provide fiber. Grains have been an essential part of nutrition for centuries. Grains have not suddenly started poisoning people.

However, the number of products labeled "gluten-free" has skyrocketed. The gluten-free market is now estimated to be around $6 billion with 20 percent of the population buying these products. Bestselling books like *Wheat Belly* and diets such as the Paleo diet, have advised against eating carbs. As a result, more people are questioning the importance of grains like wheat in their diets. Suddenly there is guilt over eating gluten.

Have you heard that wheat causes inflammation, today's wheat has more gluten, or white flours are unhealthy? Read "Wheat Belly: An Analysis of Selected Statements and Basic Theses from the Book," which debunks each of these claims.[84]

Grains provide fiber. Grains have been an essential part of nutrition for centuries. Grains have not suddenly started poisoning people.

The big questions and food myths:

- *Should I try to avoid gluten?*
- *Are grains bad for me or should I be wary of wheat?*

WHY IS WHEAT BAD WHEN QUINOA IS COOL?

As a bread maker and pasta lover, I have great respect for wheat. Between this and my farm roots, you'd think I'd have always known there are different kinds of wheat in flour traditionally used to bake bread than the wheat used for flour to make cakes. But I just assumed cake flour was more processed or refined than the standard all-purpose flour or wheat flour used in breads. There's a lot more to the story, as an Idaho wheat farmer explained.

The difference is actually the science of wheat. "Soft white wheats make the best cookies and cakes. This wheat performs well in baking cookies and cakes because soft white wheat has lower protein, which allows for products to bake with smaller bubbles at a softer texture. Hard red wheat makes better bread because a higher protein results in additional larger bubbles," said Joe Anderson, who has grown wheat for nearly 40 years in Idaho.

So what do we buy for baking at the grocery store?

Joe says all-purpose flour is likely to be mix of hard red winter and spring wheat. The difference between the two is in water absorption and the way protein (gluten) holds in air bubbles.

The value of wheat in baking is all about the protein level, which gets to the science of gluten. Gluten is actually a mix of two proteins. It is found predominately in wheat, but also in barley, rye, and spelt. Gluten is the glue that holds bread together; it's what gives bread a chewy texture.

Some books make claims that gluten has changed in wheat and leave people with the impression that wheat is a GMO. Wheat farmers like Joe take issue with those false claims. There is no GMO wheat. Studies also confirm wheat breeding has not changed the gluten content of today's wheat.[85] The protein levels have not changed.

Joe sells his wheat based upon protein levels every year, so he is familiar with wheat at a level few can understand. After nearly 40 years of experience, he knows exactly what happens to wheat's protein levels based upon how he raises his crops. He talks about research done over the last 30 years to identify what is best for baking and how new varieties have to undergo a wheat quality baking difference.

"Gluten is more a quality of protein than an actual number," says Joe, a fourth-generation farmer.

Like many wheat farmers, Joe and his brother rotate their spring and winter wheat crops with legumes such as garbanzo beans, lentils, peas for export, and sometimes malt barley. Crops are rotated for disease management (keeping the soil and plants healthy) and weed pressure across their 4,400 acres. Joe indicates wheat needs about two years to not be susceptible to disease; in other words, fields are rotated so they are not planted in the same type of wheat for two years.

Joe directly seeds wheat into the ground at planting, after using pre-emergent herbicide so the wheat can have a good start without competing against weeds. "Along with the wheat seed, the air drill planter puts down nitrogen, phosphorous, zinc, and sulfur and sometimes potassium with the wheat seed. The nutrients are used at minimal levels, determined by soil testing and base background knowledge of application rates. These are adjusted year to year if the soil didn't use the nutrients from the year prior."

IS WHEAT DRENCHED IN CHEMICALS?

"Our overage of products went from 10 percent 30 years ago to 2 percent overage now," Joe said. In other words, today's technology has allowed him use considerably fewer products, one-fifth of what was used three decades ago. "Less than 1 percent of wheat is sprayed with glyphosate just before harvest. We went four or five years without using any weed control at harvest time, but had to last year—at a very low rate—because weeds needed to be dried down or they would create problems in quality, harvesting, and grading."

He points out "Wheat kernels are protected by chaff (the casing around the actual wheat kernel). The plants are not moving the weed control to the grain head because the wheat is in the dough stage. Therefore, it's not susceptible to any weed control that does need to be sprayed."

"Farmers don't use products or GMO seeds because Monsanto makes us. It is an environmental tool that allows us to protect the soil by not disturbing it (since they are not cultivating to remove weeds) and making it susceptible to erosion."

Incidentally, there is no GMO wheat grown commercially in Canada or the United States. None! If you see food making that claim, it is marketing. And wheat hasn't been hybridized like corn because of the expense, so dismiss that claim as well if you hear it. A food truth to remember in the bread and baking aisle is that in 1950, one acre grew enough wheat for 670 loaves—today the same acre yields enough for 1,800 loaves, largely due to improved farming practices like Joe described.

WHAT ABOUT WHEAT ALLERGIES?

Wheat allergy in the entire population is under 0.5 percent. Some research shows medications may be part of the reason many people are experiencing food reactions and sensitivities to gluten. Proteins are broken down to basic peptides and amino acids by the acid in the stomach. If the stomach acid is not strong enough (either due to age or taking antacid medications), protein fragments can enter the small intestine, setting off reactions in the gut.[86]

Am I suggesting you eat a whole loaf of bread because wheat is so wonderful? No. Everything in moderation. Fiber is important to our bodies; it allows nutrients to be transported into our cells. And grains are an essential source of fiber.

But what about the obesity epidemic? Overindulge on carbs, and you're going to gain weight. The same is true if you eat too much of any type of food. But no credible study has shown gluten or wheat is the cause of obesity.

The *Dietary Guidelines* recommend making half of the grains you eat whole, so try to get some whole grains instead of a refined-grain product. When selecting bread, read the label because being brown or being labeled multigrain doesn't make bread whole grain. Look for whole-grain wheat flour to be listed as the first ingredient.

Quinoa is cool; I happen to love it. But wheat doesn't deserve to be labeled as a "bad" food because of fads and false claims. Grains and gluten are an essential part of a diet. Grains can help reduce your risk of heart disease, cancer, diabetes, and other health complications.

31. Sugar, Salt, and Everything Evil

CELEBRATING WITH SWEETS

Just as I confessed our Cheetos vacation tradition at the beginning of the book, I admit to another rather unhealthy tradition. Each August, in the midst of 90-degree humid Hoosier days and school starting, the Indiana State Fair rolls around. We take my daughter's cattle to downtown Indianapolis so she can be a part of the state 4-H dairy show (a beauty contest for cows).

> **Food Truth**
>
> Sugar, salt, and moderation are a natural part of a balanced diet.

Once we arrive, we unload several hundred pounds of hay, straw, and tack, while getting everything set up for the cattle over the span of a couple of hours. Then I ask her the key question: "What's our treat today?"

"Elephant ear," is almost always her choice on the first day. Because elephant ears evoke memories of my own days in 4-H at the Hillsdale County Fair in southern Michigan, I happily oblige. You might be wondering what an elephant ear is; it's a piece of dough stretched into a large oval, deep fried, and topped with cinnamon and sugar. The more cinnamon and sugar, the better!

After we indulge our sweet tooth, we return to the barn. We stay late to be sure all the cattle are cared for, then return before dawn the next morning. Cows have to be milked, heifers need to be washed, all of them need to be fed. When all the work is done, I again ask, "What is our treat today?"

"Funnel cake!" Also not a health food by any stretch of the imagination, but it is fun to watch them drop the cake batter out of the funnel in the deep fryer. Once it comes out, my daughter—a three-season athlete—always asks for extra powdered sugar. I secretly wonder if the extra sugar is to be sure we have to wear the white marks of our indulgence all day—funnel cakes are incredibly messy to eat.

You may be wondering why I'm writing about the copious amount of sugar we consume at the state fair. It's called transparency, and is an example of food as a celebration. I'm a mom who cherishes traditions with my daughter and hope to teach her a valuable lesson—everything in moderation.

The other side of the sugar story is us lifting 75-pound hay bales, carrying 50-pound feed bags, and handling over 1,000 pounds of cow. There's some serious calories burned on those sweaty state fair days—which helps justify our caloric intake.

A good food conscience is great, but equally valuable is celebrating life. Balance accordingly.

The big questions and food myths:

- *Shouldn't I avoid all sugar?*
- *Isn't salt bad?*

OBESITY FROM SUGAR OR REDUCED ACTIVITY?

Obesity is an epidemic in the United States. More than one-third of American adults age 20 and older are obese. According to the USDA, we went from consuming 2,388 calories/day in 1989 to 2,594 calories/day in 2009. And obesity rates climbed 12 percent between 1994 and 2010.

Why? Many people would point to sugar intake. But the numbers tell a different story. An average 433 kcal were consumed per capita from sugars in 1989. In 2009, 440 kcal on average were consumed per capita, according to International Food Information Council (IFIC). In other words, there was not a huge increase in calories consumed from sugars. Americans are eating more calories, and that overconsumption has led to rising obesity rates, increased risk for diabetes, and more cardiovascular disease.

Is it possible our weight issues in the United States and Canada are linked to less activity instead of a singular ingredient? Rather than working outside, we are sitting at our desks or lying on the couch with a screen in front of our face. As former president of the Academy of Nutrition and Dietetics, registered dietitian Marianne Edge Smith said, "Intake of sugar has not increased significantly, but our level of activity has decreased."

Dr. John Sievenpiper has stated many times that the debate on sugars is "high in opinion, low in data." His research and that of authoritative bodies have shown weight is more about total calories than it is about grams of sugars, "added" or not.[87]

Step back and define sugar. It is a simple carbohydrate. It has been consumed since the beginning of time. There are more than 20 individual, naturally found sugars, which are known as monosaccharides. Glucose, fructose, galactose, and ribose are the only four sugars absorbable into the human body.

Yet movies have been written about sugar, it is claimed to cause cancer, Food Babe chortles about sugars, and Dr. Oz offers his opinion.

In case you didn't read my personal experience with a loved one's cancer diagnosis and blaming a singular ingredient, sugar doesn't cause cancer. MD Anderson Cancer Center at the University of Texas says, "It's true that sugar feeds every cell in our body—even cancer cells. But, research shows that eating sugar doesn't necessarily lead to cancer. It's what sugar does to your waistline that can lead to cancer."[88]

"Women should have no more than six teaspoons per day (24 grams), and men should have no more than nine teaspoons per day (36 grams)," says the American Heart Association. "This equals about 100 calories for women and 150 for men."[89]

Most Americans actually eat more than double that much sugar in a day—about 22 teaspoons. That's 260 cups or 130 pounds of sugar each year.

Rather than the "sugar is bad" mantra, how about simply lessening intake? *Dietary Guidelines* for today limit intake of added sugars to less than 10 percent of total daily calories instead of the 13 to17 percent we currently consume.

My rule of thumb is to minimize soft drinks, only buy fruit in natural juices, check the Nutrition Facts Panel, read labels for hidden sugars, and keep treats to special occasions. My sweet tooth can be a huge distraction, particularly when chocolate is involved. But my drive to be healthy is stronger.

WHAT ABOUT SALT?

You would not be able to survive without salt. Sodium is an essential electrolyte; it maintains fluid balance and carries out vital functions such as regulating blood volume and nervous system activity, as well as ensuring healthy heart function and muscle contraction. If your sodium levels drop dramatically, it can lead to dizziness, severe muscle cramps, weakness, vomiting, headache, and fatigue.

Salt is not produced by the body, so sodium in nutrition allows us to function. Table salt also contains a critical element that we do not get elsewhere—iodine. Iodine is required for brain and thyroid function, and iodized table salt is recommended as the source of your sodium.[90] Sea salt, as lovely as it is to cook with, has no iodine in it.

Know that table salt is essential; it has great value, both as an electrolyte and by providing you with a source of iodine. However, too much salt or sodium is a danger.

The 2015–2020 *Dietary Guidelines* recommend consuming *less than* these levels from the "bad boys" of the bread and baking aisle:

- 10 percent of your calories per day from added sugars
- 10 percent of your calories per day from saturated fats
- 2,300 milligrams per day of sodium
- As little dietary cholesterol as possible while following a healthy eating pattern[91]

Salt is also a natural preservative, so it is often higher in canned and processed foods. For example, sodium nitrite is used to prevent botulism in cured meats. What's the secret to avoiding too much salt? Reading the label to know what products contain a lot of salt (canned soups are infamously high), adjusting your tastes to less sodium, and using products with less sodium (e.g., frozen veggies instead of canned); ask at restaurants if they could use herbs instead of salt; etc.

Salt can be deadly . . . both too much and too little. Everything in moderation.

32. Is Your Fat Better Than My Fat?

WHICH FAT IS BETTER?

Lard or butter? Coconut oil as the saving grace? Bacon as a happy food "drug." Cooking shows on TV treat saturated fats like these as though they are the star of the kitchen.

> **Food Truth**
> Fat isn't always bad.

The rest of us are left to deal with the reality of figuring out the fat puzzle, which has had conflicting messages for 50 years. Fats are kind of like politics—a lot of talk and even more opinions—with "fat causes heart attacks" on one side' and "eat all the fat you can" at the other side. Like most issues, the answer is in the middle. Moderation is key.

Did you know you need to be consuming more mono (MUFA) and polyunsaturated (PUFA) fats? IFIC's *2015 Food & Health Survey* shows that 30 percent of Americans are limiting or avoiding these fatty acids. If you want an in-depth look at fats, I recommend you read *The Big Fat Surprise* by Nina Teicholz and *Eat Fat, Get Thin* by Dr. Mark Hyman.

Registered dietitian Sally Kuzemchak writes for *Fitness* magazine. She makes recommendations such as loading up on whole food like nutrient-rich produce and whole grains, not overdoing saturated fats, considering your carbs, and indulging in a piece of dark chocolate daily in her "8 Rules to Eat By" article.[92]

Buying and cooking food requires understanding the different elements. Oils or fats are an important building block in a recipe. They have become complicated, but remember to stick close to fats created naturally. An avocado is a healthier choice than mayonnaise, and a handful of nuts is more nutritious than fried chips.

The big questions and food myths:

- *Shouldn't I avoid all fat and oil?*
- *What type of food has fat that is okay for my family?*

THE SCIENCE OF GROWING HEALTHIER OIL

There's been a tremendous amount of research done in making more natural fats, from food science labs working to reduce fat in dairy products to plant scientists breeding a better oilseed. Canola is the by-product of such science—it was developed through traditional breeding from rapeseed, while removing the undesirable characteristics. Canola oil is my favorite type of oil to cook with, so here is its story.

According to Oklahoma State University, canola oil contains just 7 percent saturated fat, compared to 15 percent for olive oil, 19 percent from peanut oil, and 12 percent for sunflower oil. Canola oil is considered the healthiest of all commonly used cooking oils. It is lowest in saturated fat and the best source of omega-3 fats of the popular oils. Canola oil, from pressed canola seed, is high in cholesterol-lowering monounsaturated fat.

Studies examining the role of canola oil in lowering blood cholesterol levels and reducing risk of coronary heart disease, cancer, diabetes, and high blood pressure have been conducted for 20 years. When used as part of a balanced diet, canola oil has been shown to lower blood cholesterol levels and have a beneficial effect on clot formation, which decreases the risk of heart disease and stroke.

Contrary to some people's thinking, canola is a crop unto itself. Canola belongs to the same family as mustard, broccoli, Brussels sprouts, and cauliflower. Canola seed is harvested from pods that are formed after those beautiful yellow flowers fade away. It's a yellow oil, usually found in between vegetable oil and corn oil.

North American farmers have been growing canola seed for over 30 years. About 1.5 million acres are grown in the United States (mostly in North Dakota). The ratio of supply versus demand of canola oil is about 1:3. The United States actually imports a great deal of canola from Canada, where 20 million acres are grown annually, according to the Canola Councils in both countries.

I met Dale Leftwich in Saskatoon a few years ago while giving a science communications workshop. Dale was an affable guy and farms in Esterhazy, Saskatchewan, with his elderly parents, wife, and daughters. They grow canola and hard spring wheat, which has gone to flour mills in the United Kingdom. He is particularly passionate about canola, which has taken him around the world. Last year he attended the Oxford Farming Conference in England and the Foreign Agricultural Organization (FAO) Conference in Italy.

He was the only North American farmer on a panel at the FAO meeting in Rome. He was joined by a cocoa farmer from Ghana, a cotton farmer from Kenya, and corn farmers from the Philippines and Argentina. The topic? They all were talking about how biotechnology (GMO) makes a huge difference in how people can farm.

"You can't hold biotechnology from the rest of the world," was Dale's perspective for the FAO.

After the four farmers were done, FAO went on record saying all of the tools in the toolbox have to be available to farmers around the world. In other words, if GMO helps solve starvation in Africa or allows food to be grown in a drought in Kenya, it needs to be available—regardless of politics.

CANOLA CARE

After growing canola for 25 years—and GMO canola for the last 15 years—Dale is well versed in the plant that's a member of the cabbage family and makes beautiful yellow flowers. "It's an incredibly elastic plant; canola can take drought favorably and respond when water comes." He also points to the economic contribution the crop makes to Canada—over $19.3 billion each year—and how it helps him take better care of his land.

"It's a broad leaf plant, so it's great for rotating with cereal crops. It changes the pressure our crops face from disease and insects," Dale explained.

Rotating is the practice of planting one type of crop after another in alternating years. Crop rotation allows the soil to replenish nutrients, along with disrupting the cycles of crop-specific diseases and the life cycle of certain weeds.

Weed control is a real issue for canola farmers because they can have their payment docked for quality. It's also why the only biotechnology (GMO) trait in canola is herbicide resistance. We begin before planting to control weeds by leaving the stubble from last year's crop on the ground. We used to plow or cultivate it and put herbicides on before planting. GMO canola actually helps us with sustainability. It allows us to reduce the number of passes through the field since we don't till the soil in advance. This is better for the soil and it reduces problems with erosion.

GMO canola also allows us to spray for exactly what is needed when we need to, but we use the minimum amount possible. Weed species, such as wild oats and millet, have adapted to farming styles of the past so changing our practices has allowed us to be more effective. We typically spray when the canola is 2 to 3 weeks old, then again 2 to 3 weeks later, which controls weeds for the rest of the season.

Canola actually ripens into a beautiful crop; it is relatively well known in the prairies for its yellow flowers. After it flowers, it's time for harvest. A farmer has to monitor this closely for a couple of different reasons. First, it's a crop that has a tendency to drop or shatter pods; research is being done on breeding a plant that can hold its pods until the seeds are mature. Second, it is 44 percent oil so it's important to be sure it's dry or it will heat up in storage after harvest.

After it leaves the farm, canola is trucked to a crushing plant, where it is turned into oil with a by-product of canola meal, which is fed to livestock. It's a great protein source because it has all of the protein from the plant—oil contains none.

One of the things to remember in the debate around GMO is the oils themselves are not genetically modified. This is true for soybeans, corn, and canola. The plant has been modified using only one gene, which is protein. Processing removes all proteins from oil. **There is no GMO in oils.** Oils from herbicide-tolerant plants are exactly the same as oil from "regular" plants.

Is canola the only healthy oil to cook with? No. ChooseMyPlate.gov shows commonly eaten oils include canola oil, corn oil, cottonseed oil, olive oil, safflower oil, soybean oil, and sunflower oil.

WHAT OILS ARE OKAY?

According the Academy of Nutrition and Dietetics' 2014 position paper on fats, "Healthy adults should consume between 20 [and] 35 percent of their calories from dietary fat, increase their consumption of omega-3 fatty acids, and limit their intake of saturated and trans fats."[93]

The USDA explains oils' inclusion in *Dietary Guidelines* "Oils are not a food group, but they do provide essential nutrients." Note that only small amounts of oils are recommended.

Most of the fats you eat should be polyunsaturated (PUFA) or monounsaturated (MUFA) fats. Oils are the major source of MUFAs and PUFAs in the diet. The PUFAs contain some fatty acids that are necessary for health—called "essential fatty acids."[94]

Oils are okay in moderation. The MUFAs and PUFAs do not raise your "bad" cholesterol (low-density lipoprotein, or LDL), and they are the major source of vitamin E in most of our diets. Just remember oils contain calories—120 calories per tablespoon.

Limit how much you consume and balance with your diet, but don't turn away from the right kinds of fats and oils. Moderation is key.

Table 7   Bread and Baking Food Truths

Food Myth	Food Truth
Farmers deplete soil in the interest of profits.	**Food Truth 15: Soil is a farm's greatest asset.** Protecting the soil for future crops—and generations—is a priority for people working the land.
Carbs are killing my diet, and no way can I eat gluten.	**Food Truth 16: Grains are an important part of your diet.** Your body needs carbohydrates and fiber to fuel your body. Grains are critical for metabolism and brain function. Gluten is the same today as it was for your grandparents; less than 0.5 percent of the population has a wheat allergy.
Avoid all sugar and salt.	**Food Truth 17: Sugar, salt, and moderation are a natural part of a balanced diet.** Sugar isn't solely responsible for cancer, and salt isn't the only reason for heart attacks. Moderation and balance are the key.
Fear fat.	**Food Truth 18: Fat isn't always bad.** The source and type of fat matter; everything in moderation. Today's oils have benefits such as lowering cholesterol and reducing the risk of stroke.

Part VII: Cereal Aisle

How do we read cereal boxes? Brands become a marketing ploy, the front of cereal boxes are billboards for crazy food claims, and products we once considered wholesome are now demonized. Check inside the cereal box for the truth!

"You can't plow a field simply by turning it over in your mind."
—Gordon B. Hinckley

33. Pardon Me, You Dropped Intellectual Property in My Food

INTELLECTUAL PROPERTY IN YOUR HAND, YARD, AND PLATE

What technology do you use every day? I'm completely an Apple girl—from my phone to my office equipment to AppleTV to my daughter's iPod. Yes, I drank their Kool-Aid and believe Steve Jobs had a brilliant mind in re-creating Apple—though I refuse to wait in line for new releases.

> **Food Truth**
> Genes are the coolest ingredient on your plate.

How many people do you know who will camp out for the latest iPhone, Apple Watch, or release from this iconic brand? They want the hottest technology in their hands as soon as it's released. Whether a business, productivity, or entertainment tool, it's technology they "have to have."

What if one of those loyal Apple fans decided to hack into the iOS (Apple's operating system) and steal intellectual property (IP)? Would they go from an Apple lover to a convicted criminal? Likely. Consider Apple's actions to protect their iOS from even the government. IP is a big deal to a business who has invested billions in developing it—and they are adamant about protecting it.

It's no different when it comes to plants. Yes, seeds are a natural plant product—you can go out to any tree or plant and find seeds. Yet, as you look at your knock-out roses, know those are patented genetics. And that beautiful flowering snowball hydrangea? It contains IP from being grafted on a tree. The sweet corn you enjoyed knowing it has been sprayed with fewer chemicals because of its genetics? Also IP.

IP does not only apply to the upper echelons of tech companies. A patent on a seed is no less important than a patent on an iPhone. There are patents on non-GMO crops like those comprising your flour, organic products, GMO seeds such as corn genetically protected against worms, and ornamental plants bred for your landscaping.

HOW CAN GENETICS BE INTELLECTUAL PROPERTY?

Check out the plant labels the next time you go to a garden center and you'll likely find a patent. Most often, it's a genetic patent because of the breeding and/

or technology involved. Keep in mind someone worked a long time and invested a lot of money to make those black petunias, grafted trees, and special-shaped shrubs.

The same is true in the food grown to make baking products and bread; there are centuries of research, improved genetics, and technology invested in the ingredients in your cereal box. Genetics used in farming and ranching (on both the crop and animal side) are intellectual property used to make more nutritious food. Examples of genetics include natural selection for a trait such as protein in dairy breeding to make better cheese, hybridization by crossing two kinds of peppers for better yield, and genetic modification by moving a bacterium gene into corn to act as a natural insecticide.

The big questions and food myths:

- *Are farmers under corporate control?*
- *How can genetics be intellectual property?*
- *Is it true that companies are suing farmers over seeds?*

ARE FARMERS UNDER CORPORATE CONTROL?

Brian Scott, a dad to two boys, grows the crops that make the products in the baking aisle. Brian raises corn, soybeans, and popcorn with his father and grandfather on a large farm. He has more data points on his tractor, iPad, and phone than most of us will see in a lifetime. He can tell you exactly what product he applied across thousands of acres, when, how it was applied, the genetics involved, and the resulting yield—and uses drones to help.

Brian openly answers pointed questions, including those about biotechnology (GMO), why farms get sued by companies, and if farms are under corporate control. He blogs and is known across social media as *The Farmer's Life*. Check out his material for a daily perspective from the farm, including his posts on CNN's *Eatrocacy* blog.

Brian has publicly shared his farm's entire biotechnology agreement, complete with his commentary:

> I've seen a lot of posts online about how corporations control farms, or farmers are slaves to "Big Ag." Some people claim that we are beholden to them and have to sign unfair contracts to be privileged enough to use their seed. They'll also claim that the contracts rope us into buying other inputs like pesticides and herbicides from the same company. We get a lot of our seed from big corporations like the "evil" Monsanto, and since Farm Aid seems to be jumping into the debate, I wanted to know what they think about some of the genetically modified crops we grow on our farm.
>
> The Farm Aid Web site poses the question "What does GE mean for family farmers?" and goes on to say "Corporate Control. Farmers who buy GE seeds must sign contracts that dictate how their crop is grown—including what chemicals to buy—and forbid them from saving seeds. This has given corporations incredible control over the production of major staple crops in America."

Let's examine this corporate control a little further and look at it from the family farm level, my farm in particular. When we buy Monsanto's biotech seeds, we sign a Technology/Stewardship Agreement (which is similar across all companies). Section 4 of the 2011 agreement I have on file covers everything the grower must agree to when purchasing these products. Here's a quick rundown of the requirements.

- If we buy or lease land that is already seeded with Monsanto technology that year, we need to abide by the contract. Makes sense to me. If I end up leasing ground in crop for some reason, I should honor the agreements it was planted with.
- Read and follow the Technology Use Guide and Insect Resistance Management/Grower Guide. Monsanto has ideas on how best to use their product. Some of it is required by the EPA to make sure farmers like me understand how to steward the technology. No big surprise there, not to mention that the guides have a ton of good agronomic information.
- Implement an Insect Resistance Management program. Shocking! Monsanto thinks controlling pests responsibly is a good idea. If you farm, insects are something you deal with no matter what type of crop you may have.
- We should only buy seed from a dealer or seed company licensed by Monsanto. I'd want to do that anyway. It's for my own good. Would you buy a brand-new home entertainment system out of the back of some guy's van parked in an alley? Me neither.
- We agree to use seed with Monsanto technology solely for planting a single commercial crop. And don't sell any to your neighbor either, it says. That's right, we can't save seed to grow the next year. Frankly I'm not interested in doing that. For the critics who are not sold on biotech crops—do you really want farmers holding onto this seed and planting it without any kind of paper trail?
- If you want to plant seed to be used as seed, you need to sign an agreement to do so with a seed company licensed by Monsanto. We do this for two different companies. In fact, we've actually worked with one company through several name changes long before biotech showed up. Why? Because we can get a premium price for the soybeans we grow that will be used as seed by other farmers next year.

We can't grow seed to be used for breeding, research, or generation of herbicide registration data. That gets back to saving seed. If we wanted to breed our own varieties, I'm sure we could get into doing that, but I look at it right now as division of labor. Seed companies are great at coming up with great products, and American farmers are the best at turning those products into a bounty of food, feed, fuel, and fiber.

See the whole piece, including a PDF of Brian's biotechnology agreement, on his blog or at my Web site. These agreements are very similar across the various companies that sell biotechnology. Although the "Monsanto is evil" belief is so prevalent, there are thousands of seeds mixed in with seeds from hundreds of other companies, small and large.

SELECTING THE RIGHT SEED FOR THE TASK

At the end of the day, it's your choice whether you support biotechnology or not, just as it's Brian's choice whether he buys GMO seed with IP and grows it on his farm. Every farmer has that choice.

With regard to IP in seed and companies suing farmers, Brian said, "I don't have any major issues with IP as it relates to plants. An individual or company put a lot of time, effort, and dollars into breeding a crop or ornamental plant to fit a certain task."

He points out that most farmers don't want to be crop breeders. "Give us the best seeds for our soils, developed by people who are absolute experts in their profession. We'll take those seeds and make them perform."

In other words, it is a farmer's choice to select their genetics—and spend money on IP or not—based on their farm. Conditions change from season to season and area to area.

"As far as companies like Monsanto suing farmers for breach of contract, I don't see a problem there either. You signed a contract, and you broke it. Don't like the terms of the contract? Find seed that doesn't require that step.

"The idea that seed companies are pushing small farms out of business and are constantly suing farmers is blown way out of proportion. A lot of the misinformation on this topic occurs online where the people complaining are posting from computers and mobile devices packed with patents of their own."

34. The Demonization of the Corn Stalk

SWEET CORN OR FIELD CORN?

Meg, a friend and fellow professional speaker from suburban Chicago, visited our farm with her daughter, Frankie, on a beautiful blue-sky summer weekend. Frankie soon started asking a flurry of questions, including, "What is that growing in the field? Isn't that sweet corn?" Frankie had correctly identified it as corn, but then we had a 30-minute discussion about the differences in types of corn with these city friends.

> **Food Truth**
>
> Corn is tasty—and healthy—for animals and people.

"See how most of the corn is a bunch taller and has bigger stalks than other corn? That's field corn," I explained. Most of the time in the Midwest, you see field corn. Field corn is not sweet corn. It is grown as livestock feed, use in human food, or for ethanol. Field corn comprises 99 percent of the corn crop in the United States. Humans can eat it, but field corn is starchy and bland, without the sugar contents found in sweet corn. There's nothing "wrong" with field corn—and the fields are not filled with poisons—but field corn just doesn't taste good until it is processed into a product.

Unfortunately, corn has been vilified in recent years, from movies being made about how corn is poisonous, farmers being forced to grow corn, and how such a monoculture crop is destroying the environment.

There's no need to demonize the corn stalk, though—corn is healthy for both animals and people. Corn is an important part of a diet, whether it is sweet corn in the vegetable case, corn meal in the baking aisle, or white corn in tortilla chips. Corn is also essential to livestock as an energy source; in other words, it helps to feed livestock to produce meat, milk, and eggs. That's actually where the majority of corn goes: 34 percent of field corn is used as livestock feed, according to the USDA.

The big questions and food myths:

- *Isn't high-fructose corn syrup (HFCS) awful?*
- *How can corn be safe with the claims about being bad for cows and kids?*
- *Isn't all corn GMO?*

HIGH-FRUCTOSE CORN SYRUP

As you grab a box of corn flakes, you're likely not thinking that corn has been consumed for 7,000 years. It has evolved from a plant that had kernels more like wheat into the present-day tall green stalk that the USDA reports being grown across 88 million acres in the United States.

According to some claims, it's the green giant grown to poison us all, leading to obesity, higher food prices, learning disabilities, and lead poisoning. It's the reason why this is the only food truth that singles out a specific commodity. I don't grow corn, but I certainly know the value of it in feed for my animals, on my own plate, and in my grocery cart.

I'll refer you back to the meat case chapter for why animals need corn. It has to do with energy, feed palatability and a properly functioning rumen in cattle.

You're likely thinking about sugar when you go down the cereal aisle, so what about high-fructose corn syrup (HFCS)? Is it making us fat? Obesity is caused by eating more calories than you burn. HFCS does contribute calories, but there is no scientific evidence that the sweetener uniquely contributes to obesity or diabetes. USDA data shows that consumption of HFCS has recently been declining, whereas obesity and diabetes rates continue to rise. Obesity is also rising globally, even though HFCS is fairly limited in other countries.

Why was HFCS ever made? The USDA first listed HFCS as safe for food use back in 1983, but the use started in the 1970s when the food industry was looking for alternatives to sugar. HFCS is a less expensive, relatively low-calorie way to sweeten processed foods, and is very similar to sugar.

Sugar is from either sugar cane (most production has been driven out of North America because of production costs) or sugar beets (which are now GMO to better resist virus, fungus, herbicides, and nematodes). Table sugar is 50 percent fructose and 50 percent glucose.

HFCS is syrup made from corn starch. There are two forms of HFCS; one has 42 percent fructose and 58 percent glucose, and the other is 55 percent fructose and 45 percent glucose. Both have 16 calories per teaspoon. In other words, HFCS is nearly identical to sugar. Contrary to what you may have been led to believe, table sugar, HFCS, and honey are all digested and metabolized similarly according to tests.[95]

HFCS is a simple, cheap way to give consumers the taste they desire. Food manufacturers use it because it is known for providing sweetness; enhancing fruit, citrus, and spice flavors; and preserving food and texture.

But marketing smear tactics create fear around HFCS. The corn growers and the sugar growers ended up in court because "The Sugar Association has made numerous false and misleading representations that processed sugar is different from high fructose corn syrup in ways that are beneficial to consumers' health. The Sugar Association preys on consumers' fears," by falsely representing that HFCS causes a number of health issues, including obesity, "while at the same time creating a health halo for processed sugar."[96]

It saddens me to see those in agriculture attack each other. However, I agree that vilifying one kind of added sweetener is not right, nor is it ethical to insinuate that one ingredient uniquely contributes to obesity and other health problems when science contradicts that.

The type of sweetener is not the problem; it's the amount of sweetener consumed. If you're drinking a liter of sugar-laden soda and eating three pastries, that's a lot of calories. AND advises consumers that they can safely enjoy nutritive sweeteners when they are consumed as part of an overall diet that meets government recommendations.[97]

Should you try to avoid HFCS or not? That is completely up to you; just know that it meets FDA guidelines to be a natural sweetener, as it does not contain artificial or synthetic ingredients or color additives. I don't believe it's the demon many have claimed, but I do moderate intake of all sweeteners for my family when possible.

IS THERE CHOICE IN GROWING CORN OR
IS IT LIKE KING CORN SAYS?

Not all farmers choose to farm the same way. Enter Justin and Jennifer Dammam from Iowa, a pair of dynamic 30-somethings who farm over 2,400 acres. I met Jennifer at a leadership training I gave in 2009. "Farming is our families' legacy. We have been farming here for 115 years and we are passionate about growing crops and livestock to feed and fuel the world," said Justin.

Recently, they have chosen to plant non-GMO corn. "The consumer, in my opinion, has sent a clear message that a certain percentage of our customers are willing to pay for non-GMO products. We never really thought we'd go back to non-GMO, but it has seemed to gain a lot of traction with consumers," Jennifer explained.

Justin and Jennifer contract all of their specialty corn with a plant 20 miles away, which means their farming has some controls attached.

"Yes, we do have some limitations. We are limited on seed selection; there are only certain brands of seed and hybrids we are allowed to plant based on milling quality. Currently where we are contracted they only have one brand we can use, so we have very few options to choose from." That shows one of the challenges for farmers who contract; some of their options are removed.

"We are not allowed more than 1 percent GMO in our crop. We cannot use glyphosate as a weed killer and since the corn is food grade, we spend more dollars on our inputs to keep the quality of the grain protected. For example, the fields have fungicides and insecticides applied by plane to keep pests from damaging the crop. The non-GMO is more susceptible to disease and insects," said Jennifer.

As the Dammanns both agree, there is no singular "right way" to farm. It's about making a choice that is right for the family business and being able to manage their farm accordingly. For example, non-GMO crops take more insecticides and fungicides.

"If we were to not use pesticides, yields would be much lower, fieldwork would be exponentially more labor intense—and we could not feed as many people with the acres we have to farm. Yields can be unpredictable if the weather is not ideal and the chemicals to combat corn borer and root worm cost more."

A variety of products are made from their corn. "There are literally thousands of products from the corn and soybeans we grow, but the ones that are most popular are tortilla chips, corn flakes, cereals, tacos, and cooking oils. There are also popular products outside of the grocery store including SmartStrand Corn Carpet (which we have in our house), ethanol gasoline, adhesives, dry wall, many cosmetics, varnish, some plastic containers and even some window cleaners," Jennifer said.

Jennifer and Justin have gone to where the market is, as more major brands are claiming to be GMO-free. They are fortunate to have a processor closely to contract with to purchase their specialty grain. Specialty markets are just that—specialized to a need or an area. In order for a farm to make it financially viable to change to a specific practice or product, it's often under a contract.

Aside from the business part of it, the Dammanns, who have two cute kids, summed up what so many farmers feel about growing crops: "It is more than just a job, it is a way of life and we take pride in watching a nurtured seed placed in soil, sprout and become a healthy mature plant. Farmers love what we do and take what we do to heart."

Yes, there is a lot of pride in farming. Farming is a very personal act. It's difficult for a farmer to separate false claims and questions about their farming practices from who they are. In other words, when the corn stalk is demonized, so is the farmer who grows it.

35. Is the Environment Sacrificed for Profitability?

CAN EFFICIENT AND ENVIRONMENTAL PRACTICES COEXIST?

You'd have to look hard to find a better model of efficiency than farming. Today's farmers and ranchers produce 262 percent more food with 2 percent fewer inputs compared to 1950, according to the American Farm Bureau Federation.

> **Food Truth**
>
> Sustainability is complex and essential to family businesses.

As Wisconsin corn and soybean farmer Kevin Hoyer said, "Sustainability is multipronged. It's about improving upon what you have by positively influencing environmental, economic, and society factors."

Farmers are price takers, not price makers. In nearly every segment, they are told what their price will be—regardless of weather, cost of input products, and regulatory requirements. Farmers need to make enough in the end to support their family or it is not a sustainable business.

In 2015 the USDA counted 18,000 fewer farms compared to the previous year and a million fewer acres of farmland. They estimated the total number of U.S. farms at 2.07 million and the total number of farm acres at 912 million. The average farm size is three acres bigger than a year prior, at 441 acres.

Why the continued downward slide in the number of farms? There are many factors—from lower prices at the farm gate, an aging farm population, increased regulatory concerns, and environmental pressures. Does this mean that efficiency is more important than environmental sustainability? Do farmers make economic decisions without regard to environmental consequence? As several farmers explained throughout this book, sustainability includes care for both the environment and economics. It's a complex equation, one that includes changing practices and increasing scrutiny.

The big questions and food myths:

• *Aren't farmers just in it for the profit?*
• *Isn't it more sustainable to go back to old-time farming?*

DRONES AS A SUSTAINABILITY TOOL?

Most people wouldn't say fainting goats and miniature horses go hand in hand with drones (unmanned aerial vehicles, or UAVs), but they do for northern Illinois farmer Matt Boucher. As a dad to three kids not quite in their teenage years, he prioritizes spending time with his family and making memories with his wife, two daughters, and one son. Matt believes drones help him do that and farm more sustainably. Drones help Matt make better use of his time, target inputs specifically where they are needed, and identify problems across his 900 acres of corn, soybean, and wheat fields.

Matt is an early adopter and a leader in using drones on farms for agronomic purposes (he also sells them to other farmers). In other words, he is using them to make healthier plants and soil.

"It improves scouting (the evaluation of bug, weed, and disease pressure in a crop) tremendously. I can fly a field in 10 minutes instead of walking it for hours and hours. My accuracy is far better with a drone than when I walked every few rows and may have missed something," Matt said.

How does this help the environment?

The drone actually takes various pictures as it flies across the field and combines them all into one image on an SD file. Farmers like Matt can review the image and see what is happening across his entire field to determine what needs to be done. With the use of GPS technology, the SD file can be loaded right into the applicator (sprayer) to determine exactly where to spray the bug control (pesticide) or fungicide or fertilizer, based upon the way the plants look. Matt points out that there may be 20 acres in one corner of the field needing treatment and 30 acres in another area—and that's all that gets treated. It's a whole lot more precise—and better for the environment—than the older practice of treating an entire field.

Drones aren't widely accepted by a lot of farms, but most new technology isn't until it's proven.

Matt operates with the philosophy, "There's always something different that makes us better."

"The technology we're using in our drones now has been used in planes. It's fairly new technology; we're flying a lot lower and get a lot more detail. Our knowhow of using that tech is evolving, as is how to react. It's all in its infancy." He went on to liken drones to desktop computers 25 years ago. There will be a better one two weeks later.

However, drones have to make financial sense—a kit costs anywhere from $1,000 to $17,000. "Looking at it from a crop scouting side, it's the amount of time you save. If I fly every acre one time, it only costs me $2/acre, which is only half a bushel of corn. It also allows me to target and use inputs more efficiently, which are expensive—particularly insecticides and fungicides."

When asked what he really wishes people understood about people who farm products found in the cereal aisle, Matt was quick to respond, "We are trying to use few inputs to produce as much or more food products. We are not out dousing things. We are trying to do the best job we can."

TECHNOLOGY HELPS THE ENVIRONMENT AND WILDLIFE

Matt plants both GMO and non-GMO corn. He questions which is better because he has to spray the non-GMO more, but pays more for the GMO seed.

Certain ground is better for non-GMO. "Everybody has to make that decision on their own—it's a mistake to make a blanket statement without understanding the whole picture."

A recent Purdue University study[98] that looked at whether banning GMOs would negatively affect the environment showed higher food prices, a significant boost in greenhouse gas emissions due to land use change, and major loss of forest and pasture land if GMOs in the United States were banned. Given the position many environmental activists have taken against GMOs, this is an interesting finding. "Commodity prices would rise with lower crop yields without GMO. Corn prices would increase as much as 28 percent and soybeans as much as 22 percent. All of that means your food prices would rise 1 to 2 percent, or $14 billion to $24 billion per year," concluded the Purdue study.

One may be able to afford higher food costs and believe that a GMO ban is worth any price. But what about the single mom already struggling to pay for food? If such a ban was instituted, wouldn't it be unsustainable due to consequences in both the environment and grocery budgets?

The environmental impacts of today's farming practices are not taken lightly by the families who grow your food. Ninety-nine percent of farmers say they care about environmental practices, and nearly 75 percent of consumers are concerned about the use of pesticides and insecticides used in farming.

As stated by Steven Savage, a plant pathologist, in *Forbes* magazine, "In 2014, to have raised all U.S. crops as organic would have required 109 million more acres of land, an area equivalent to ALL the parkland and wild land areas in the lower 48 states, or 1.8 times as much as all the urban land in the nation."[99]

THE FINANCIAL ASPECT OF SUSTAINABILITY

Sustainability shouldn't only be about the land, water, and air—or going backwards to practices from when "times were simpler." Sustainability is also about utilizing technology to help the environment and strengthen the economy on family farms, for as a farm thrives, so does the community in which it operates.

A recent study in Minnesota[100] showed a farmer spends $960,000 in their greater community each year on average. Over the course of 40 years farming or ranching, this adds up to $38 million. Is this because farmers are rich? Not likely, but they do support local businesses and are fiercely loyal once trust is earned.

How does a farmer spend nearly a million dollars annually in their greater community?

- 16.9 percent on interest and leases
- 16.4 percent on seed, fertilizer, and chemicals
- 14.5 percent on capital purchases
- 10.6 percent on purchased feed
- 10.0 percent on family living
- 7.6 percent on feeder livestock and custom work

- 7.0 percent on fuel and repairs
- 4.2 percent on hired labor
- 4.2 percent on other livestock expenses
- 3.5 percent on general farm expenses
- 3.0 percent on other crop expenses
- 2.1 percent on taxes and utilities

How does community spending add up? The study shows 1,287 farmers spend over $1.2 *billion* dollars in a community in one year alone.[101]

Those dollars not only provide for schools and roads, but contribute to the long-term viability of the community. The figures may vary from state to state, but the contributions of farms and ranches to a community are significant. A sustainable farm not only cares for the environment but also tends to their business across generations, which, in turn, support a vibrant community.

36. What Is Pecksniffery?

WHEN BELIEFS AND BEHAVIORS DIFFER

"Seth Pecksniff, a character with a holier-than-thou attitude in Charles Dickens's 1844 novel *Martin Chuzzlewit*, was no angel, though he certainly tried to pass himself off as one. Pecksniff liked to preach morality and brag about his own virtue, but in reality he was a deceptive rascal who would use any means to advance his own selfish interests." according to *Merriam-Webster*.

> **Food Truth**
> Hypocrisy happens in food, health, and nutrition.

Why do you need to know this? Pecksniffery has been used as a synonym for hypocrite, apparently since 1949. How does that relate to food? Well, finding a way to point out the inconsistent actions we take around issues related to food, health, and nutrition has cost me a lot of worry. But a farm-mom friend in Illinois gave me the perfect word from her thesaurus: pecksniffery.

Pecksniffery is a way of saying that we want to hold certain beliefs around what is right in food, health, and nutrition, yet we sometimes behave differently. For example, I believe in eating healthy, but then stress drives me to chocolate. I intend to do the right thing, but my actions do not always align with my belief.

Inconsistent behavior happens all over the grocery store, including in the cereal aisle. Have you bought any organic Fruit Loops lately? How about some natural Cocoa Puffs? Why, when General Mills made a GMO-free Cheerios, did sales not increase at all?

If we pause and become aware of our choices, we're likely to find hypocrisy on our plate, in our cart, and across food labels.

Case in point: potatoes. Potato grower John Halverson points to the sales of potatoes as an example of consumers spending their dollars differently than they say they will when surveyed about food choices: "Consumers constantly say they are looking at healthy attributes, but sales of fresh potatoes continue to shrink while sale of chips and fries grow at record pace."

Let's face it; we all want to believe we'll buy "healthy" food, but then reality strikes. Or in this case, the potato chip crinkles. At the deli, in a restaurant, or a fairgrounds food booth, a French fry reaches out and grabs you. We may want to believe we'll buy more "whole" food like a baked potato, but the numbers don't lie about America's preference for fried food.

The same goes with issues like GMOs. One of the reasons I've extensively covered this contentious issue is because of the hypocrisy involved. Is GMO evil in your grocery cart but miraculous if it saves a little girl's life? Is GMO good if it can cure blindness through golden rice but wrong if used to keep worms out of sweet corn?

Canadian farmer Dale Leftwich talks about the medical value of GMOs. Not because of the crops he grows in his fields north of the border, but because it's far more personal to him. Dale has a daughter who was diagnosed with diabetes at age seven. "Life is better because of a stable source of insulin due to a GMO process with bacteria producing insulin. There's an abundant source of consistent, cost-effective insulin due to GMO," he explained.

Is it possible emotionalism has clouded our thinking on issues like GMO, how meat is raised, and "big" agriculture? Is it possible we are practicing pecksniffery?

The big questions and food myths:

- *Shouldn't I be more concerned, not less, about issues related to food?*
- *Would someone just tell me what is "the right thing to do"?*

TRANSPARENCY AROUND THE FOOD PLATE

The call for transparency from farmers and ranchers has been heard loud and clear. It is one of the fundamental underpinnings of this book to expose how your food really is being raised by the people who are doing it; I've tried to share a variety of transparent stories from farms and ranches. But where do conscious choices with the food buyer begin?

For example, is it inconsistent to be worrying about all-purpose flour that has been bleached while drinking chlorine-treated water? How about fussing over about the trace amounts of bleach used to sanitize apples but not being concerned with getting your hair treated by mostly unregulated chemicals applied directly to your scalp? The same standards should apply.

Personally, I'm fine with white flour used in baking—it just makes a better product in some recipes. I also know water grows bacteria and parasites, so a bit of chlorination to keep it healthy makes sense me. And bleach or dye my hair—that's every woman's secret, but I'm also fine with that practice. Those are my standards. What are yours?

Knowing your family's ethical, nutritional, environmental, and social standards results in consistent beliefs and behaviors. What is right for you may not be right for your next-door neighbor—and that's okay. The point is that you spent time finding your own standards around food.

Contradictory beliefs and behavior also happen in our view on weight gain. The IFIC Foundation's *2014 Food & Health Survey* studied the trend blaming sugar as the source of calories most responsible for weight gain. Forty percent of respondents said that sugars and carbohydrates were most responsible for weight gain, compared to 29 percent who said all sources contribute equally; 15 percent weren't sure.

What about the lack of exercise balancing out the caloric intake? "I meant to walk for 30 minutes, but there was a work deadline and a soccer game." Isn't there a certain amount of incongruence in blaming a single ingredient for weight gain if one's behavior is inconsistent with a healthy lifestyle?

ABOUT THAT PERFECTLY GREEN LAWN . . .

Do you strive for the best yard in the neighborhood, without a bug or weed in sight or use an exterminator to get rid of those pesky ants? How many chemicals are applied to the yard where your pets live, your kids play, and your family walks through on a daily basis?

The National Academy of Science points to lawn use as a significant part of what they say is the "pesticide problem." According to the EPA, homeowners use 10 times more pesticides per acre than farmers do, although the farmer uses pesticides more widely.[102] The Web site shows a riding lawnmower pollutes as much in one hour as does driving a typical automobile for 45 miles.

Is it inconsistent for a homeowner with a bleach-cleaned, bug-free house and perfect yard to only buy organic?

ABOUT YOUR FOOD CHOICES . . .

At some level, our behaviors differ from our beliefs. We don't intend to practice pecksniffery, but the pressure to "do the right thing" with food seems to be driving guilt in the grocery.

Some brands try to tell you what your standards need to be in the interest of profit, such as Whole Foods. The Austin-based company is unquestionably "big business" with 91,000 workers in 437 stores worldwide and $15 billion in sales in 2015 according to their Web site. If your standards align with Whole Foods and you can afford to shop there, please do so. Just know those standards aren't all about wholesome food, but include financial incentives. It's hypocritical to suggest otherwise.

Marketing capitalizes on your guilt. That guilt evolves into double standards. Double standards are taken advantage of by brands. Food shaming happens. It's a vicious cycle, one that has made food buying far more emotional than it needs to be. Doing the "right" thing is your choice—and only your choice.

It's time to stop letting others manipulate your food choices. Differing beliefs and behavior flies in the face of simplifying your food choices. Ask questions when a claim doesn't sound quite right. If you find food being an emotionally led decision, pause to ask why.

You are doing your best for your family. Know your standards. Stick to them. Call yourself and others out for pecksniffery—preferably with kindness.

Table 8   Cereal Aisle Food Truths

Food Myth	Food Truth
A seed is natural; it can't be intellectual property.	**Food Truth 10: Genes are the coolest ingredient on your plate.** Corn, oats, and soybeans are all products of the intellectual property of genetic improvement.
Corn is bad.	**Food Truth 19: Corn is tasty—and healthy—for animals and people.** Sweet corn for you and field corn for livestock is an important energy source.
Mass grain production hurts the environment.	**Food Truth 12: Sustainability is complex and essential to family businesses.** Environmental audits, technology, and family business survival skills all make up a model that is sustainable for generations.
Buying and eating behavior always aligns with beliefs.	**Food Truth 20: Hypocrisy happens in food, health, and nutrition.** We all want to believe we would buy healthy food and exercise on plan, but do we really? Transparency needs to happen on all sides of the plate.

Part VIII: Snacks and Convenience Foods

Are there more kinds of fats today than there were choices in crackers 20 years ago? Take a look at the issues in snacks and convenience, including label claims, the long-term impacts of your nutrition cases, and short-term permission to accept convenience as reality. Leave the food shaming behind as you explore this aisle.

"Food, in the end, in our own tradition, is something holy. It's not about nutrients and calories. It's about sharing. It's about honesty. It's about identity."

—Louise Fresco

37. The Reality of Convenience

HARRIED PARENT GUILT

Do you ever feel like an Olympian juggler? Finish up a major project to meet a work deadline. Get kids fed after school. Shuttle to basketball, then piano. Pick up dry cleaning. Run to grocery store. Don't forget the dog food. Get to the baseball game.

> **Food Truth**
>
> Convenience is reality; it's not always wrong or right.

And then it's time to feed everyone. Yikes, there's no time for that, but they are screaming "we are hungryyyy." Grab some fruit to go, throw veggies in a snack bag, and hit a drive thru to get your family fed in between activities. Then just breathe—they are happily eating.

Some believe they can't stop at fast food joints. That's a choice. Others believe anything pre-cut in produce is wrong. That's a choice. Another may avoid canned or frozen fruit or vegetables. That's a choice. One choice is not right while the others are wrong.

I believe today's harried parents need permission to STOP THE GUILT. If buying a bag of pre-cut apples at McDonald's is the best you can do to get fruit in your kiddo one evening, so be it. Likewise, if you live in snow in the winter, frozen and canned fruit are better than going without. If using frozen vegetables allows you enough time to cook a meal, you are doing the right thing.

Food guilt is alive and well, even in the small town I live in. As I was enjoying a glass of wine with a group of friends one evening, the conversation turned to guilt at the grocery. I was surprised to find even the most independent moms fall prey to food shaming and worry about being judged by what's in their cart.

One friend fussed about being judged by processed foods like pizza bites in her cart since one of her sons struggles with weight. Another worried what it looks like if cross-fit people see her cart has anything but fresh ingredients with the "right" label. A third stressed about people judging her if she has any processed foods in her cart.

Let me be crystal clear; your grocery cart is your business. No one else's. Convenience is sometimes necessary—do not let others tell you what is right or wrong for your family. Only you know your reality.

The big questions and food myths:

- *Isn't it bad to eat convenience food?*
- *Is it always wrong to buy processed foods?*
- *What am I eating when in a rush?*

WHERE ARE YOU ON THE CONVENIENCE SCALE?

Food choices often depend on nutritional priorities, family traditions, and health perspective. For example, I enjoy going out to special restaurants on occasion. I believe in cooking, though it usually involves ingredients that are frozen or canned to save time. My friend and his son eat out at least five nights a week. He doesn't know how to cook and believes it makes a mess.

Where are you on the convenience scale? Do you go to the high end of the scale—eating out on a daily basis and buying all packaged food that can be thrown in the oven? Or are you on the scale's low end, rarely going to a restaurant or using any packaged products?

No answer is perfect. You may need to purchase frozen meals for your kids staying after school for a musical. They can have a salad the next day—the world won't end. Likewise, if you are higher on the convenience scale, you could consider grabbing a bag of carrots instead of Cheetos. The reality of convenience without health costs lies in balance and moderation.

FOOD FORECASTING

Jessica Crandall of Denver, Colorado, is a registered dietitian, a personal trainer, and a diabetes educator—a busy lady who understands the necessity of convenience.

"Being busy is a big part of people's everyday life. Recognizing it allows you to be prepared for it. I advise 'food forecasting'—know what you're going to be eating next. You can have health and convenience together—you can bring snacks with you, such as apples and almonds."

But fast food or quick-serve restaurants are often a part of getting busy families fed, so how do we best choose when that becomes a necessity?

Jessica explains, "Balance is really important. Look over the menu first and think about what you want versus what you need. Are there modifications you can make? For example, can you get fruit or salad instead of fries? Do you really need all the dressings and condiments?" She also raises the ultimate issue for anyone concerned with weight and nutrition while dealing with a crazy calendar: Are you committed to your goals or just interested in them?"

That's life—and you likely have the same challenge. There are ways to simplify cooking and plan ahead. But you have to be committed in order to do it. I'm not going to proclaim highly processed foods are okay all the time, but I also believe that a 14-year-old boy learning to bake a pizza is better than eating two orders of

French fries. Likewise, it's valuable for a five year-old girl to help grow veggies she can enjoy on her dinner plate.

REDUCING COOKING TIME

One of the simplest ways to minimize cooking time is to use "convenience" items like canned and frozen fruits and vegetables. The American Academy of Pediatrics (AAP), as well as the American Medical Association (AMA), the American Cancer Society, AND, the Institute of Food Technologists, the American Institute of Nutrition, and the American Society for Clinical Nutrition want parents to feed their children *more*, not less, of a variety of fruits and vegetables.

These organizations don't say only eat a certain kind of produce. They did not say only raw produce. Rather, the recommendation is to bring more fruits and vegetables into your family for better health. Sometimes convenience is a part of that.

Studies conducted by the University of Georgia (UGA) and the University of California-Davis (UC Davis) show frozen fruits and vegetables are as rich in nutrients, and often more so, than fresh-stored produce. Specifically, the "market basket" study by UGA found the amounts of vitamin A, vitamin C, and foliates in several frozen fruits and vegetables are actually greater than their fresh-stored counterparts. Similarly, the UC Davis study found frozen fruits and vegetables are nutritionally equivalent to fresh-stored produce.[103]

Canned foods can also be an affordable option to get your nutrition. Just watch the nutrition panel for sodium and added sugar. Whether it's canned beans as a side dish, canned artichokes for a casserole, lentil soup, or fruit in natural juices, canned and frozen foods are a quick way to get nutrition.

A friend once told me if every meal was balanced, the world would wobble. As much as I believe in nutritious meals, life happens. Give yourself permission that some days are better than others; convenience doesn't mean you are not doing your best for your family. It means you're living!

38. Balancing Choice on the Plate and the Farm

WHO DECIDES THEIR IDENTITY?

As a business owner, I value the freedom to make choices about who I'll work with and how we will work together. I have been fortunate that this has included Fortune 100 companies and entrepreneurial start-ups. I choose not to work with organizations that don't prioritize ethics, and I will not work with any group that wants me to include their marketing in my speeches. My choice is to operate my business to best serve the people interested in farm and food.

> **Food Truth**
>
> Choice on the farm and choice on the plate involve a balancing act.

Farmers and ranchers also value choice. This is called freedom to operate; the ability to make decisions best suited for our family, land, and animals. And since independence is one of the strongest traits among farmers and ranchers, we don't take kindly to people telling us how to take care of our land or animals.

And as a mother, I am particularly protective of my choice on how to feed my family. Aren't you? I've made nutritional choices for my daughter since the day she was conceived and am slowly turning those over to her as she learns the value of nutrition. I don't need any government agency, farmer, or media limiting my choices on my family's plate. You likely feel the same about your choices.

So which is more important? Choice on the plate or choice on the farm? A farm family makes one choice. You may make another choice. One is not wrong and the other right; choices around the food plate should be symbiotic. Food is about sharing, honesty, and identity. It's your choice of what is right for your family.

The big questions and food myths:

- *Shouldn't all farmers be only organic?*
- *Is it true that farmers choose to farm one way or the other—and that's the only way?*

ONE FOOT IN ORGANICS, THE OTHER IN CONVENTIONAL FARMING

Did you know an organic farm could have 1,100 acres of land, raise seed for a company, and grow 7,000 conventionally raised hogs annually? Meet Jon and Carolyn Olson from Minnesota, who just had their farm recognized as a century farm. The house they live in and land they farm was purchased by Jonathan's great grandfather in 1913 and registered as Fairview Farms for $0.50 a year later. The couple runs the farm, along with one full-time employee and their youngest daughter, who works for the farm on summer breaks from college.

The Olsons have a unique operation between their certified organic grains and conventionally raised hogs. Carolyn is quite vocal in her support of ALL kinds of agriculture. "I believe that every farmer needs to find what works for them and their farm. Organic agriculture is not for everyone, and neither is dairy farming, or pig farming, or vegetable growing. Diversity in agriculture should be celebrated."

They raise corn, soybeans, and wheat on a pretty strict rotation to help them manage weeds. Carolyn says, "Occasionally we will have a field of barley and field peas, or oats, or triticale on small grain ground if we are asked to raise them for seed."

> Seeds are the lifeblood of any crop, so seed companies often contract with farmers to raise crops for seed.
>
> Our soybeans and wheat are raised for seed for the Albert Lea Seed House in Albert Lea, Minnesota. Our farm has been producing seed certified through the Minnesota Crop Improvement Association since the 1940s. The corn is sold either for human consumption (vodka, corn flakes, etc.), or animal feed. The soybeans and wheat that are not used for seed are sold for animal feed, or the wheat may be used for flour or other wheat-based products in prepackaged foods.
>
> When we decided to transition to organic, part of our conversations revolved around the pig barns. Should we continue to finish pigs conventionally? We didn't have the pasture space or the proper barn style to raise pigs organically, and we knew we needed a source of animal manure for our crops, so we made the decision to continue finishing pigs as we always have. Some wonder how we can raise conventional pigs and grow organic crops, but I don't see why this has to be an either/or thing.

In the words of an organic and conventional farmer, it's a choice, and one that even farmers don't always agree on. Unfortunately, marketing on food with claims about the "right way" way to grow food is deepening that divide.

Matt and Anne Burkholder in Nebraska are another couple exemplifying both choice on the farm and on the food plate. "We have a diversified farm in order to supply a variety of markets and customers. Historically, our farm was 100 percent traditional crops but we got into the organic markets in 2006. Organic farming, if managed well, can bring in quite a bit more profit with a market that is not typically as volatile as conventional markets because it is a niche market."

In addition to previously having a beef feedlot, they have 600 acres of grass pasture, 1,800 acres of conventional alfalfa, 1,400 acres of organic alfalfa, 500 acres of conventional corn, 500 acres of organic corn, 60 acres of conventional soybeans, and 160 acres of conventional oat hay—plus a few horses, cats, and dogs. Anne indicates the blend allows for the family farm's financial sustainability to grow both organic and conventional crops.

She was quick to add, "They each come with a set of positives and negatives. Using a blend of organic and conventional on our farm allows us to diversify to best meet a variety of challenges. Judiciously using resources is important to us and we can optimize that by growing a blend of both traditional and organic crops."

Finding the right type of operation is different for every farmer and depends on their skillset, available resources, market, type of land, and personal values. One is not right and the other wrong.

Make your choices based on your own standards—just as farmers make those choices for their business.

39. Cheap Food Will Cost You More Later

EXERCISE IS A PRIVILEGE

Spinning is my therapy. Not spinning yarn or even a tale, but spinning on a bike. I go twice a week to sweat like mad while seeing how fast I can make my legs fly to obnoxiously loud rock music while my beloved teacher, Val, yells. It's an awesome workout to combat stress, burn calories, and build endurance. It's also one of the few intense exercise classes I am still allowed to do. I was born with abnormal knee structure and had surgery on both of them when I was 15. I refused to let them limit me as a long-distance runner in track in high school and ran harder than ever the year after the surgeries.

> **Food Truth**
> Pay less now, and pay more later in your health and the environment.

When I was 24, my doctor in California told me that I'd have a double knee replacement by the time I was 50 if I didn't stop high-impact aerobics or give up running. Major knee surgery a few years ago left me flat on my back for weeks. It taught me exercise is a privilege and health is an investment. Sure, it's easier to sit on the couch with potato chips and ignore nutrition, but what you invest in your body today pays off years later. That is true in both food and exercise.

The big questions and food myths:

- *I deserve this treat, so why not indulge?*
- *My choice today won't really matter in 30 years, will it?*
- *How can I get my kids to eat healthier?*

INVESTING IN YOURSELF

"Disease states, such as diabetes, high blood pressure, and obesity, are progressive. Unless you are taking preventative measures, the disease is going to start taking control of your life," points out AND spokesperson Jessica, who addresses convenience and nutrition in Chapter 37. "Every day is an opportunity to take preventative measure—a chance for you be mindful of what you're consuming, your portion and your activity level."

She likens it to your retirement plan; many people do not start thinking about it until they get older. "And then people realize it's not just about longevity, but also the quality of life. They want to be healthy and active, but also be with their grandkids—not just sitting on the sidelines. Investing in yourself is a daily commitment, not just when you retire."

Nutritional choices are a major contributor to health problems in the United States, along with the associated healthcare costs. The conversation turned to childhood obesity and the fact that obesity in kids is growing about 1 percent each year.

CONNECTING NUTRITION WITH CHILDREN (AND STUBBORN ADULTS)

How can we get through to kids about the importance of nutrition?

"Take a pause and reflect on how you want to teach them. What do good, healthy behaviors look like? You need to model that behavior for them and encourage active participation in meals," Jessica explained. She offered these tips to engage kids (and perhaps some stubborn adults) in nutrition:

- Have dinner at the table five times per week—it's really important.
- Reduce their screen time—either eliminate it one day a week or cut down daily.
- Watch calories and nutrition content (or lack of it) in small things like drinks and snacks.
- Involve your kids in grocery shopping.
- Have them plate their own food.
- Involve them in cooking.
- Find out what's important to them and what would spur commitment.

Learn about and talk to kids at the grocery store about why nutrition matters to their athletic and academic performance, how they can take good food to school, and what to look for on food packages. This may take herculean acts of patience, but will likely produce long-term results for their health.

MORE LIFE THROUGH HEALTHY BEHAVIORS

Jessica says, "Food does not make memories; people rarely remember what they had for dinner unless it was a special occasion. Life makes a lot of great memories. In order to have more life, you have to have healthy behaviors."

One of the fastest-growing trends is for food retailers to involve dietitians. Leah McGrath is a registered dietitian who has worked for Ingles Markets in North Carolina for 16 years. She suggested checking your supermarket's Web site in their health and nutrition section to see if a retail store dietitian is available. "It's very chain or retailer dependent. Some chains offer medical nutrition therapy for counseling on obesity, diabetes, high blood pressure, etc. Other stores are doing group activities, such as store tours and cooking demonstrations."

Whether you work with a dietitian or not, here's the bottom line. It may be cheaper to buy Coke instead of milk for your kids today, but the long-term health consequences will be expensive. It's faster to grab water bottles than fill your own travel bottle, but what are the consequences in the landfill? It may be easier to grab a highly processed, fully cooked meal, but if you're not evaluating nutrient balance in your diet, your life won't be easier in the long term.

Healthy behavior requires discipline. I choose more life. You decide what is right for you long-term.

40. Are They Sneaky Snacks or Are We Label Illiterate?

THE FEAR OF DIHYDROGEN MONOXIDE

Have you heard about dihydrogen monoxide? You likely have it in your car, have sent it to school with your child, and keep it in your refrigerator. You likely used nearly 170 bottles of it last year.

> **Food Truth**
>
> Food is an amazing science from farm to table.

According to the Web site DHMO.org, "Dihydrogen Monoxide (DHMO) is a colorless and odorless chemical compound, also referred to by some as Dihydrogen Oxide, Hydrogen Hydroxide, Hydronium Hydroxide, or simply Hydric acid. Its basis is the highly reactive hydroxyl radical, a species shown to mutate DNA, denature proteins, disrupt cell membranes, and chemically alter critical neurotransmitters. The atomic components of DHMO are found in a number of caustic, explosive and poisonous compounds such as Sulfuric Acid, Nitroglycerine and Ethyl Alcohol."

One complaint on the Web site was "I've been seeing on the Internet stories about a sandwich shop using a chemical called DHMO (dihydrogen monoxide) in their bread that is supposed to be an industrial solvent used in fire-retardant materials and is waste from nuclear power plants; it is supposed to be toxic. I was wondering the truth behind this rumor and if you guys could investigate?"

This was actually the subject of a science fair project by a 14-year-old in Idaho Falls back in 1997, entitled "How Gullible Are We?" He made the news because of how he presented warnings about the dangers of dihydrogen monoxide and asking people what (if anything) should be done about the chemical. The story has since been used in science education to encourage critical thinking.[104]

Why the call for critical thinking? Dihydrogen monoxide is water. Two (di) hydrogen molecules plus one (mono) oxygen or oxide is H_2O.

Yes, water. The scientific name makes it sound scary. "If you can't pronounce it, you shouldn't eat it," is a common claim. However, there is a reason chemical and scientific names are being used in food ingredients. It's called consistency. Otherwise, one company could, instead of using "sodium bicarbonate" on a food label, list "all natural fairy fluff" while another writes "baking soda." Scientific names help us standardize food packages rather than having more claims to woo and confuse food buyers.

What if you can't pronounce jalapeño, quinoa, gyro, or prosciutto? Does that mean you shouldn't eat them? Should you never consume something unfamiliar to you?

Rather than fearing science in food, there is reason to celebrate it. Whether you can pronounce a scientific term involved with food is irrelevant to its nutritional value. If you love food, embrace the science in it. Science should be the grounding force in the highly emotional discussion around food.

The big questions and food myths:

- *What's hiding in my snacks?*
- *How do I know if ingredients are really safe?*
- *Why put additives in food?*

A CONTINUUM OF LEARNING

"As the daughter of an agricultural research scientist, I came to understand at an early age agriculture (as well as all other professions) is a continuum of learning. As we develop better methods or products, perhaps we were not 'wrong' until we made old practices obsolete. We live in a society that wallows in perceived or created controversy which distracts us, or creates a barrier, to honest dialogue and learning from each other and moving forward in societal and scientific inquiry, testing, and change when necessary," was the comment made on Facebook by Donna Rocker from Georgia.

Perhaps not what you want to think about when munching on snacks, but useful nonetheless. If you're picking up a box of crackers, do you really know the ingredients the same way as when you pick up an apple to munch on—or just know there is controversy? Do you have a continuum of learning when it comes to what's in your food?

Rule number one to avoid scary processed food ingredients: eat what you know—food that still resembles its initial state. In other words, avoid highly processed snacks when you can and grab some snow peas, a handful of almonds, banana, jerky, or a handful of cranberries.

Rule number two: Realize snacks will be a part of your diet and make conscious choices about what you put in your body. The reality is people eat processed food and some may point a finger at "hidden" ingredients.

WHAT ARE THOSE ADDITIVES ANYHOW?

Remember: additives help preserve the freshness, safety, taste, and appearance of foods. Had any rancid fat lately? You'd know it by the smell if you had— antioxidants prevent fats and oils from becoming rancid. Like peanut butter as a power snack? We do, too, but it's gross when it separates into solids and liquids. Emulsifiers stop peanut butter from separating. Like to have canned fruit that is firm and resembles its natural color? Additives help that to happen.

Argue about additives and preservatives—food ingredients that may sound really strange—if you wish, but know they play important functions. They are particularly important to shelf life and reducing food waste.

Even organic foods contain additives. There are currently 29 additives approved for use in organic foods. Without additives, bread becomes stale very quickly, fatty foods turn rancid, and most tinned fruits and vegetables lose their firmness and color.[105]

The FDA, which has the primary responsibility for determining if an additive is safe, maintains a list of over 3,000 ingredients in its database "Everything Added to Food in the United States," many of which we use at home every day (e.g., sugar, baking soda, salt, vanilla, yeast, spices, and colors).[106]

WHY ADDITIVES?

Why have additives in food? These are the three key reasons, according to the FDA:

1. *Maintain and improve freshness:* Preservatives slow spoilage caused by mold, air, bacteria, fungi, or yeast. This helps with quality and prevents foodborne illness, such as botulism.
2. *Improve or maintain nutritional value:* Vitamins and minerals are added to many foods to make up for what's lacking in your diet or is lost in processing. This has helped reduce malnutrition in the United States and worldwide.
3. *Improve taste, texture, and appearance:* Spices, natural and artificial flavors, and sweeteners are added to improve taste. Food colors help with appearance, and leavening agents allow baked goods to rise. Emulsifiers, stabilizers, and thickeners give foods the expected texture and consistency.

The FDA Web site says the safety of a substance and whether it should be approved are determined by:

1. The composition and properties of the substance
2. The amount that would be typically consumed

3. Immediate and long-term health effects
4. Various safety factors

There is a built-in safety margin when additives are evaluated so that the levels of use that gain approval are much lower than what could have adverse effects.

"Recognize we are always making some sort of compromise. Given the times we live in, we are going to have to make some compromises that some food will be processed. For example, if you want to have a frozen TV dinner—there are things that have to be done to that meal to make it acceptable and palatable. If you don't want to eat food with ingredients like that, you have to make compromise in other parts of your life and take more time," said John Coupland, a food scientist at Penn State University, in a phone conversation.

Compromise in food science makes sense—as does understanding the consequences if one additive is removed from food. What's going to happen if we don't use that ingredient? Will there be more food waste if stabilizers and preservatives—which many consumers think of as "chemicals"—are removed from food? What will it do to availability and cost of a product?

Check a package for food ingredients. The IFIC's brochure on additives is helpful and available at http://www.foodinsight.org/Food_Ingredients_Colors.

Evaluate content and context before drawing conclusions, whether it's an ingredient list on frozen vegetables or pizza rolls. There's science in both, though one is likely a healthier choice. You decide.

Table 9   Snacks and Convenience Food Truths

Food Myth	Food Truth
Eating convenient or processed food is unhealthy.	**Food Truth 21: Convenience is reality; it's not always wrong or right.** Quick food is sometimes the only option, and guilt shouldn't be a part of the food choices you make for your family.
Consumers are right, farmers are wrong. Farmers are right, consumers are wrong.	**Food Truth 22: Choice on the farm and choice on the plate involve a balancing act.** Democracy brings choice on both sides of the food plate. What you choose to feed your family is equally important as how a farmer chooses to farm. One should not trump the other.
I don't have the money to buy good food.	**Food Truth 23: Pay less now, and pay more later in your health.** Both are a long-term investment. Soda may be cheaper than milk, but offers no nutritional value.
If I can't pronounce it, I shouldn't eat it.	**Food Truth 13: Food is an amazing science from farm to table.** There is no need to fear your food. Science benefits you, helps the environment, and makes better food.

Part IX: Deli and Foodservice

Harried schedules and less interest in cooking have made the deli one of the fastest-growing grocery trends. The deli has grown beyond fried chicken and cupcakes to a smorgasbord for the eyes and taste buds. Is the deli fresher, better for you, or simply higher priced? And what about fast food?

"People who love to eat are always the best people."

—Julia Child

41. Whose Hands Have Been in Your Food?

WHAT'S IN A HAND?

Do you know the most common source of food contamination? Think it's from animals? During processing? At the grocery store? Nope. Look closer.

> **Food Truth**
>
> Food safety starts on the farm and ends in your kitchen.

Your hands are the most common source of food contamination. Well, to be clear, not just your hands—everyone's. Poor hand hygiene accounts for an overwhelming number of foodborne illness outbreaks. The quality and frequency of hand washing bottoms out with high school–aged individuals, showing only 8 percent of males washed their hands after using the bathroom![107] Consider who makes up a large number of foodservice industry workers to know why education in the workplace becomes a critical tool to keep restaurant patrons safe. In order to protect consumers and prevent bad press, teaching hygiene in foodservice is a priority. It's not necessarily the foods themselves that are making people sick, but rather how they are being handled.

Produce accounts for over half of all illnesses reported, with norovirus as the culprit bug.[108] Luckily norovirus, typically mistaken as stomach flu, is generally not deadly and is easily preventable. When preparing food at home, uncut produce is best for food safety. Precut, washed, and packaged vegetables pose the most risk as they are handled far more than whole, fresh vegetables.

The IFIC's *2015 Food and Health Survey* showed the top foodborne illness is no longer the top food safety concern among Americans. Thirty-six percent of Americans ranked "chemicals in food" as the most important food safety issue. That's a 13 percent increase over the year prior, which shows unscientific marketing is scaring people more than the reality of foodborne illness.

"The risks posed by pesticides in food pale in comparison to the risks from foodborne illness," said Carl Winter, a food toxicologist and vice chair of the Department of Food Science and Technology at the University of California at Davis.[109]

The big questions and food myths:

- *How do I know the food is safe when I eat out?*
- *What is the best way to avoid foodborne illness?*

FOOD WITH INTEGRITY OR ILLNESS?

What is a case study in food safety concerns in restaurants? Chipotle, whose Web site claims, "Since we opened the first Chipotle restaurant more than 22 years ago, we have served fresh, wholesome ingredients prepared using classic cooking techniques. It's always been a top priority to make sure that our delicious food is safe to eat."

Really? Let's take a look at the burrito chain's history of foodborne illness in 2015. The last one sickened 151 people in Boston in December 2015 and led to the closing of that location. The other documented foodborne illnesses in 2015 were:

- Seattle—*E. coli* O157:H7, July 2015, five sick people, source unknown.
- Simi Valley, California—Norovirus, August 2015, 234 people, source was sick employee.
- Minnesota—Salmonella newport, August and September 2015, 64 sick people, source was tomatoes but it is not known at what point in the field-to-fork chain the pathogen was introduced.
- Nine states—*E. coli* O26, began October 2015 and declared over February 1, 2916, 55 sick people, source unknown, states involved were California, Delaware, Illinois, Kentucky, Maryland, Minnesota, New York, Ohio, Oregon, Pennsylvania, and Washington.
- Three states—*E. coli* O26, began December 2015 declared over February 1, 2016, five sick people, source unknown, states involved were Kansas, Oklahoma, and Nebraska.[110]

According to Food Safety News, "Chipotle faces more than 100 civil claims by outbreak victims and their families . . . Stockholders also have filed at least two federal court cases seeking class action status. The civil suits claim Chipotle violated the Securities Exchange Act by making false and/or misleading statements. The stockholders contend:

- Chipotle's quality controls were not in compliance with applicable consumer and workplace safety regulations.
- Chipotle's quality controls were inadequate to safeguard consumer and employee health, and as a result of the foregoing, Chipotle's public statements were materially false and misleading at all relevant times."

Let's talk about pork raised without any antibiotics—it doesn't always make the most sense if the animal is sick, nor is it always the safest method. Thus why Chipotle couldn't find enough pork in the United States and imported it from the

United Kingdom. This raises a lot of questions when the brand claims to "support local farmers," particularly coupled with their history of importing beef from Australia.

The complicated system of modern food production and FDA and USDA regulations are there for a reason. To keep our food safe. Whether you love or hate the government, it is the only system we have and is certainly more trustworthy than a brand claim.

Where you eat is up to you. Some go for the coolest names and claims, whereas others are all about the comfort food. That's personal choice. If I see food not being properly handled in the deli or an unclean restaurant, I leave because of the risk for foodborne illness. If history shows that a restaurant has had a foodborne illness problem, it's important to understand why (with apologies again on the grossness factor)—sometimes it's from deer poop on spinach and other times it's because workers don't wash their hands.

Ask yourself if a brand's claims are ethical. If so, eat with joy—after you wash your hands—and hope the people who prepared your food do the same.

42. Just Because You Can't Pronounce It Doesn't Mean It's Bad for You

PRONUNCIATION OF A FOOD INGREDIENT DOES NOT DEFINE NUTRITION

Would you eat an egg with "amino acids, phenylalanine, octadecenoic acid, sugars, colors E160c and E306, flavors phenyl acetaldehyde and acetone—also contains benzene and sulfur" on the ingredient label?

> **Food Truth**
>
> The media isn't the best source of information about food.

What about blueberries labeled with the following ingredients: sugars made up of 48 percent fructose, fatty acids like linoleic acid, flavors ethyl ethanolate and hydroxyl linalool, and colors E163a and E163e?

Food elitist and author Michael Pollan often promotes "Don't eat what you can't pronounce." I beg to differ—I love blueberries and keep them stocked in both of my freezers. Eggs are a nutritional building block for my family. I may trip over my tongue while trying to pronounce all of those ingredients, but why should a journalist be telling me what to eat?

Every ingredient listed earlier for blueberries and eggs is a chemical that naturally occurs. Australian chemistry teacher James Kennedy wanted to dispel a myth that chemicals are bad for us so he created an ingredient list for natural products. He also noted that DNA could be listed, but he left it off for brevity's sake.[111]

As the *Business Insider* article featuring Kennedy noted, "Marketers often feed off consumers' concerns that 'man-made' chemicals are bad. But the fact is that all foods (and everything around us) are made up of chemicals, whether they occur in nature or are made in a lab."

Science does not make for sexy sound bites, but it's a whole lot more reliable than a journalistic opinion. Turn to science, not away from it.

The big questions and food myths:

- *There are so many problems in agriculture, can I really trust it?*
- *I shouldn't eat what I can't pronounce, should I?*

WHAT ABOUT MONOCULTURE CONCERNS IN THE MEDIA?

Iida Ruishalme, a Finn living in Switzerland, who is a mix of a cell biologist, science communicator, and fiction writer, blogs at *Thoughtscapism*. Iida provided another example that elitists like to use as an argument against modern agriculture: monoculture is the "great evil" in American agriculture. She wrote, "A major problem with these arguments is that monoculture as a concept is very broad. Before we specify which type and degree of monoculture is the issue, we don't really know what we are talking about. What is monoculture, and what is it not?"

One example is a vineyard meeting the criteria for popular opinion about monoculture—the same product grown in the same space year after year. While visiting Australia, one of my fondest memories is the vineyards—including a Shiraz vineyard that was over a century old. The same goes for olive orchards I visited in Italy. If that's monoculture, I'll sign up any day—those are tasty products from healthy plants standing the test of time.

"What people often may be referring to when they name monoculture as the problem is the practice of growing the same crop on the same field year after year after year, that is, monocropping," wrote Iida.

As farmers have explained throughout this book, few monocrop, many use cover crops, and most rotate their crops. "Using crop rotations means that the farmer alternates the type of plant grown on one land area—the opposite of what is often meant when referring to 'monoculture.' Crop rotations have several advantages. They help avoid build-up of pathogens and pests that favor one type of crop, and they can improve soil structure and composition of nutrients by alternating deep-rooted and shallow-rooted plants, or including nitrogen-fixing legume crops, for instance."[112]

As Oklahoma farmer Curtis Vap told me, "I don't farm the same way my dad did. He didn't farm the same way my grandfather did. For the most part we do the best we can with the knowledge and technology we have at the time. Can we look back and see what we could have done better? Sure we can. But if someone criticizes our practices today, first I have to ask, do they truly know a better way or is their agenda their own enrichment and self-interest?"

DO YOU KNOW WHAT'S IN YOUR MEDIA?

Self-interest should not replace science. Leah McGrath, a dietitian for a regional supermarket chain based in North Carolina, started her career as an officer and dietitian in the Army, then a district director for WIC (Women, Infants, and Children) in South Carolina. Her dad's type 2 diabetes deepened her personal interest in the intersection of health and food. "My point of view is to scan for science. I am a big proponent of evidence-based information and like to remind people that the fad or trend likely doesn't have any science to back it up. Even when I'm presenting information to consumers in the store, I try to assure whatever I'm presenting is evidence and science based—not just trying to sell products."

Understanding science can be difficult because people face information overload. "People are bombarded with social media, TV, etc. Look for resources that are unbiased and see what their agenda is. Follow the money trail—what is the motive of the individual or site trying to persuade you? Are they trying to sell you a product or create fear?" she advised.

Case in point: Food Babe. Vani Hari, the Food Babe's real name, shows no scientific credentials, education in dietetics, or professional background in food on her Web site. She started eating differently and lost weight, and then blogged about it. She now sells products ranging from meal plans to juicing blenders to the "Food Babe Way" and specializes in creating fear about food through her "investigations."

While I agree we could all better understand what is in our food, I do not find it ethical to bully food companies or encourage an "army" to do so when there is no scientific evidence involved. In her words, "Companies have no choice but to respond to us and improve the quality of their products." She proudly lists her fear mongering on her site, such as strong-arming Chick-fil-A into announcing a plan to use antibiotic-free chickens back in 2011, convincing Kraft to change their mac and cheese recipe, and inflaming people around Starbucks' Pumpkin Spice Latte.

Hari is clearly gifted at creating headlines, but may I suggest a more accurate one would be "What's your agenda?" I find it difficult to believe an online name selling products has a better understanding of food ingredients than food scientists, microbiologists, and the FDA. There's an extensive approval process and database of ingredients.

WILL LUNCHMEAT GIVE YOU CANCER?

One of the most popular stops at the deli is for lunchmeat. Recent media headlines have given people pause about whether they should skip lunchmeat in fear it causes cancer. Should we also skip sunlight, working the third shift, or drinking alcohol? All have the same classification of causing cancer as lunchmeat.

The International Agency for Research on Cancer (IARC), a part of the World Health Organization, released findings in October 2015 showing there was a relationship between cancer and meat. They labeled processed meat a "probable carcinogen" and red meat a "possible carcinogen."

According to Janeal Yancey, the meat scientist from the University of Arkansas, the report did not say processed meat is going to give you cancer. "IARC looked at a body of evidence and were just looking for relationship. The report showed there is a relationship—the same as there is with hormone therapy, sunlight, and alcohol. It did not say lunchmeat or red meat would cause cancer, which is a very complicated disease. Of the 900 things they've looked at, they've only found that one does not cause cancer. There are too many good things about processed meats."

This perspective on balance and moderation was offered by Dr. Julie Jones, Professor Emerita of Foods and Nutrition at St. Catherine University: "Too little exercise is another problem that increases colon cancer. Too many calories is the other big promoter of colon cancer. Matching calories to needs, right sizing meat portions, and eating the recommended foods from all the food groups is a boring but proven strategy. Colon cancer rates will only be addressed if consumers start to eat a diet that has the right stuff—the right number of calories, the right amount of dietary fiber, fruits and vegetables, and dairy, substances shown to be protective against colon cancer—eat the recommended size servings of meat and exercise."[113]

LET'S GET BACK TO COMMON SENSE AND CRITICAL THINKING

Scientific names can be scary. Chemical names can create concern unless you've taken high school chemistry. In fact, food ingredients can be downright overwhelming. But media claims should not negate the nutrition or value an ingredient or farming practice brings to your food plate. Stand on science.

So what are you supposed to believe? My hope is that you'll turn toward farmers and ranchers if the question is about a particular practice in food production. If a concern is about nutrition, find a registered dietitian who should be making science-based recommendations versus their personal opinion. If it's about an additive or processing technique, look up a food scientist or an authoritative (credentialed) food science book or organization Web page.

Find experts who use science and do not sensationalize. Focus first on the source, considering who is presenting the information, what their credentials are, and what their incentive is for presenting the information. Don't rely on sensationalized videos, one-sided journalism, or celebrities for your food information.

WHAT QUESTIONS DO I ASK?

These are some of the most common questions found:

- *How is my food being produced?* Ask a farmer; they can give you great detail about today's farming, how practices are done, and why.

- *I have dietetic concerns, what should I be eating?* Rely on a registered dietitian; AND requires them to make science-based recommendations rather than on personal opinion about production style.
- *What about the article I read citing science?* Check the science, check the source, check for common sense. Critical thinking is your friend.

43. We're Not Crossing Frogs and Corn

GIRL SCOUTS AND GMOS

Girl Scouts of America refused to bend to activist tactics attacking the use of GMO ingredients in their cookies in a high-pressure online campaign. GSA supports science with answers in their Web site FAQ. Their position directly aligns with their work encouraging STEM (science education) for girls, rather than being swayed by social pressure about ingredients that a second grader couldn't read, as the campaign claimed.[114] "At the current time, there are

> **Food Truth**
> Genes are the coolest ingredient on your plate.

genetically modified agricultural crops (GMOs) in Girl Scout Cookies . . . it is important to note that there is worldwide scientific support for the safety of currently commercialized ingredients derived from genetically modified agricultural crops."

The organization even cites sources, teaching their members the value of credible scientific information. "The World Health Organization, the Food and Agriculture Organization of the United Nations, the U.S. National Academy of Sciences, and the American Medical Association all share this assessment."

Then they took the issue to a more global scale, again a teachable moment for their members. "In addition, in the future, GMOs may offer a way to help feed an ever-increasing world population."[115] Today, 28 countries, including 20 developing countries, all plant GMO crops—and the number is growing because of benefits to consumers, farmers, the environment, and medicine.

There is a great deal of fiction around genetics in food, as noted by the founder of Greenpeace, Patrick Moore, who stated, "Environmental activists scare the world's population against biotechnology based on fiction. . . . So, the campaign is basically that genetically modified foods result in reduced use of pesticides, reduced soil erosion, increased productivity, improved healthy nutrition, no known damage to anything; so, let's ban it. It is based solely on superstition. There is no basis to do it."[116]

The big questions and food myths:

- *What exactly is a GMO?*
- *Why mess with genes?*
- *Has enough research really been done?*

THE GORE OF GMO

Paul Hodgen, who holds a PhD in agronomy, the husband of a meat scientist and a dad of four, farms in Indiana with his mom and dad. They manage several thousand acres of corn and soybeans across a few counties, carefully monitoring their costs, soil health, inputs, and yields with the help of a couple employees.

"Farmers are better stewards of the environment than what people actually give us credit for. We have to take care of the soil because that is where my livelihood comes from. Without the soil, I can't raise a crop." Paul has colorful field maps illustrating the kind of seed planted in each part of the field and what products had been applied to each area—more detail than most people have in their doctor's file!

I watched Paul operate his equipment from his iPad, adjust the satellite automatically steering a 15-ton combine, and monitor the yield of the field he was combining. "This technology allows us to be more precise with our applications and inputs, from the number of seeds per acre that I am planting, to the amount of fertilizer in specific parts across each field. It also allows me to document what I am doing and depending on the season, see if that was the proper things to do or not. I have a software program that will allow me to analyze my yield. That's kind of the score card from an agronomic standpoint of how well I am doing after producing corn as efficiently as possible."

"Technology also gives me a plan for each hybrid. The biotechnology (GMO) and insect protection that comes with GMO products allows me to use less pesticides, particularly very harsh pesticides. Now I don't have to be exposed to as harsh of chemicals to raise the corn crop efficiently and safely for consumers."

Paul explains biotechnology in this way:

"The biotechnology part is really fascinating science. It's complicated science, but the concept is pretty simple. We find something in one plant and discover a trait or something in one species of plant or bacterium and say hey, we need this in corn. So then they isolate that gene. Sometimes they run it through a model plant to see if it performs and does what they think it will and then try it in corn or beans. After that, they start the crossing process to get into commercial production."

How is that different than hybridization? Does that biotechnology alter the plant?

Paul responded, "Natural breeding selection is the same thing we've been doing since man first realized if we paid attention and improved plant production, genetics can improve yield. As our understanding of genetics in all species has improved—human, livestock, plants—our ability to transfer specific genes to address disease response, or yield, has improved. GMOs are just another tool in the box that allows us to keep increasing yields and keep food prices low."

Here's what the World Health Organization says on why genetically modified (GM) foods are produced.

> GM foods are developed—and marketed—because there is some perceived advantage either to the producer or consumer of these foods, such as a lower price, greater benefit (in terms of durability or nutritional value) or both.
>
> Resistance against insects is achieved by incorporating into the food plant the gene for toxin production from the bacterium *Bacillus thuringiensis* (Bt). This toxin is currently used as a conventional insecticide in agriculture and is safe for human consumption. GM crops that inherently produce this toxin have been shown to require lower quantities of insecticides in specific situations, e.g. where pest pressure is high. Virus resistance is achieved through the introduction of a gene from certain viruses which cause disease in plants. Virus resistance makes plants less susceptible to diseases caused by such viruses, resulting in higher crop yields.
>
> Herbicide tolerance is achieved through the introduction of a gene from a bacterium conveying resistance to some herbicides. In situations where weed pressure is high, the use of such crops has resulted in a reduction in the quantity of the herbicides use.[117]

The science can be tough to get through, but this is what you need to know. It takes around $150 million to bring a genetically modified product to market. Decades of research are required. Genetic engineering has the ability to improve nutrition, reduce the use of pesticides, allow for crops to grow in drought-stricken regions of the world, and grow food as an answer to malnutrition. Yet, emotions rule the conversation around genetics in food.

You decide where you stand on genetic modification when you shop the snack and convenience aisle. I choose science and applaud genetics in keeping my grocery bill low.

GENETICS IMPROVE YOUR GROCERIES

Beef cattle have been bred to have less fat in the meat, dairy cattle have higher-protein milk, and chickens and turkeys have larger breasts, all because of genetic selection. And genetic manipulation also brought us seedless grapes and seedless watermelons, as well as a rice genetically modified to provide vitamin A and help prevent 500,000 cases of blindness and up to 2 million deaths each year. The list goes on.

When did all of this genetic manipulation start? Plants and animals have been selectively bred for centuries to amplify desirable traits while minimizing less desirable ones. The first genetically modified crop was 8,000 years ago, designed by nature with bacteria in soil as the engineers. Scientists at the International Potato Center in Lima, Peru, found genes from *Agrobacterium* in 291 sweet potato varieties, including ones grown in the United States, Indonesia, China, parts of South America, and Africa.[118] In other words, genes were transferred from bacteria to sweet potatoes in evolutionary times. This is technically called transgenics (the transfer of genetics), which sounds a bit nicer than genetically modified organism.

No one is sticking a plant, ear of corn, or fruit with a syringe or crossing them with frogs (yes, I have had questions to that effect). This is actually revolutionary science that may someday help humans solve diseases like cancer.

History shows genetic modification, gene editing, transgenics, hybridization, gene silencing, and newer breeding techniques have proven benefits. Among those benefits:

- Increased consumer convenience: seedless fruits and apples and potatoes that don't brown
- More affordable food: more production per acre or animal decreases costs
- Greater medical options: today's insulin is a direct result of transgenics
- Better nutrition with leaner, higher protein: lower-fat meats, higher-protein milk
- Solutions to malnutrition: vitamin A in rice, research on other foods like sorghum
- Improved opportunity for small-scale farmers: drought-resistant, hardier crops and animals
- Reduced carbon emissions: fewer passes through the field, higher production
- Decreased use of insecticides: corn, eggplants, and others resistant to bugs don't need sprayed
- Improved animal welfare: selection for disposition, calving ease, and polled traits
- Greater preservation of biodiversity: less land required with higher production

When you are waiting to be served chicken at a fast food restaurant or salad from the grocery store deli, you probably are not thinking about genetics. However, a whole lot of DNA is on your plate—when you hear about gene editing, transgenics, and even genetic modifications, consider the history and their possibilities to bring better health, food, and nutrition.

44. Everything in Moderation

THE PAIN OF PAYING FOR FOOD

Last week I was at the grocery store and heard a person in the next aisle complaining about the food prices, "Those darned farmers and the government bailing them out with subsidies and crop insurance."

"Nearly 80 percent of the 'farm bill' is for food assistance programs" was on the tip of my tongue, but I noticed

> **Food Truth**
> Food costs are a shared concern.

the person behind me was ready to pay with a Supplemental Nutrition Assistance Program card—the food stamp program. I didn't have time to go over to the person swearing about farmers, so I bit my tongue. If she understood the economic story of food production, she would not be blaming or complaining about farmers and ranchers.

Few understand the risk farmers and ranchers live with daily. Everything they work so hard for can be gone in 24 hours. A hail storm can destroy a wheat field ready to be harvested, flooding can leave a field unable to be planted, a disease can kill a barnful of turkeys that have $100,000 feed in them, a drought can bring end to a century-old ranch. Just because a farm or ranch has invested $500,000 in raising food does not mean there is a guaranteed return—or stability.

Friends tell me they find food prices frustrating. "All I really want is great-tasting, affordable, healthy food. Why does it have to cost so much?"

The politics and propaganda increasing the price of food are a frustrating problem for all of us. According to the 2015 Science and Food Survey, released October 2015 by the Chicago Council on Global Affairs, 92 percent of Americans consider it "somewhat important" to "very important" that food be affordable, followed by the 91 percent who felt the same way about nutrition.

The big questions and food myths:

- *Aren't farmers subsidized and getting rich?*
- *Does the government pay farmers so they have it easy?*

THE BOTTOM LINE OF FOOD PRODUCTION

Farmers and ranchers share the concern of rising food costs. They spend their days thinking about the cost of food production. As an example, a fifth-generation farmer who farms several thousand acres in central Nebraska shared his estimates on what it costs to raise food today.

Equipment (used) at $1,252,000 total or $250,000 annually:

- Planter: around $6,000 per row with a standard 24-row planter=$150,000
- Combine: $300,000–$400,000 depending on horsepower, capacity, etc.
- Head for combine: $60,000–$70,000 each for a corn head and a wheat/soybean head
- Trailer for combine head: $7,000 trailer for each to move from field to field
- Tractor: $300,000–$400,000 for 300+ horsepower needs
- Self-propelled sprayer: $200,000
- Grain cart: $30,000–$60,000 depending on accessories
- Semi: $20,000–$90,000
- Semi-trailer: $30,000
- Auto steer, variable rate, other precision tools @ $80,000

Seeds @ $156,000 for 2,000 acres:

- Corn: $180 per bag (non-GMO) to about $300 per bag (every GMO trait possible)
- Each bag has 80,000 seeds and plants 2.5 acres. 1,000 acres=$96,000
- Soybeans: $55–$65 per bag, plants one acre. 1,000 acres @ $60,000

Inputs @ $548,000 for 2,000 acres:

- Corn @ $331,000 for 1,000 acres
  - $181/acre for chemical, fertilizer, and insurance
  - 150/acre for planting, spraying, and harvest costs
- Soybeans @ $217,000 for 1,000 acres
  - $67/acre for chemical, fertilizer, and insurance
  - $150/acre for planting, spraying, and harvest costs
    (Using the University of Nebraska crop budgets for pivot irrigated, traited crops)

Land @ $600,000 for 2,000 rented acres ($300/acre)

Bottom line: It costs $1,634,000 to raise 2,000 acres of corn, soybeans, and popcorn! I used median costs, assumed a five-year simple depreciation on equipment, and rented ground instead of owned. There are also no family living expenses, labor, diesel, or salary calculated into this scenario, which is essentially a $1.6 million bet against Mother Nature.

"Farmers are heavily subsidized" or "The government pays farmers" is a common misperception. Crops are now supported through crop insurance, which the farmer can choose to buy or not. In Indiana, this costs about $25/acre *if* the farmer chooses it. An Indiana farmer shared his insurance claims average about $100/acre for corn and wheat and $0 for beans across a drought year (2014) and one with too much water (2015). If insurance was purchased, it would add another $95,000 income (after taking the insurance costs out).What's the expected profitability of the scenario laid out? If the farm raised the 2014 USDA average of 177 bushels of corn on each of their 1,000 acres and received $3.75/bushel, they would sell their corn for $663,750. The 1,000 acres of soybeans, using the 2014 USDA average of 47 bushels/acre, sold at $9.25/bushel would bring in $446,500.

The total income for this 2,000 acre farm? $1,110,200.

$1.1 million sounds like a lot of money, right? When the expenses are added in, this calculates to a $523,750 *loss*. A farmer loses half a million dollars to grow 2,000 acres? Yes, under the current market conditions. Admittedly, corn and soybean farming was considerably more profitable around 2010 because of global demand for corn, but this downward cycle is fairly consistent in the agricultural marketplace. It is a high-risk business that is getting riskier.

IS COMMODITY AGRICULTURE TO BLAME?

Some question "commodity" agriculture and feel farmers should just switch to another crop or grow a variety of animals. But consider the equipment costs just noted, the expertise highlighted throughout this book, and the complexity of the agrifood system. Those are factors whether a family has corn, cattle, or cantaloupe. Does it really seem as simple as you once thought for a farmer to change from growing wheat to quinoa?

Expenses, insurance, and support programs vary by what is grown, by where it is grown, and by whom it is grown. There are small farms making a very healthy profit, just as there are large farms and ranches doing the same. There are also ranches in the middle run by all ages, races, and both men and women. However, the reality is farming and ranching is one of the riskiest businesses in our universe. It is a very tough business and one that has changed dramatically in the last decade.

The USDA counted 18,000 fewer farms in 2014 as compared to 201, and a million fewer acres of farmland. The average age of a farmer today is 57 years old, which means food production is undergoing a massive generational shift. Being such a capital-intensive business, farming and ranching is tough to get launched and established.

The 2,000 acres I used in the example is actually not that large of farm today, primarily due to the significant risk outlined earlier. A family farm may support an older generation, a daughter's family, and a son who wants to come home to farm, so the size needs to increase in order to support family members coming home to the business. The bottom line improves with more acres or head to spread out costs, so most farms expand, diversify, or find a niche market to control their risk.

GROWING FOOD IS EXPENSIVE

At the risk of getting too economical in the last section of the book, here's a quick sampling of the expenses associated with raising food, from ice cream to pork sandwiches to salads from the deli.

- $800,000 in capital investment in equipment and building space to milk 240 cows with robots.[119]
- Farmland costs $6,000–$18,000 per acre, depending on state or province, with rates higher on either coast. Fifty acres of farmland is lost to development every hour in the United States.
- Hogs may cost $50/head to feed, which adds up to $5 million in feed costs for 100,000 head.
- Fruits and vegetables require the highest dollar inputs; it is not unusual to spend $10,000 an acre on produce.
- Additional paperwork to meet regulations requires additional labor, increasing overhead by $20,000–$30,000 annually.

Keep in mind prices received for any given product do not necessarily rise when inputs do. If fuel goes up from $2.25 to $2.85 at the pump, you notice a little jump in what you pay at the gas tank. A farmer buying 10,000 gallons of diesel sees a $0.60 rise in fuel prices, which adds up to $6,000. Unlike at the gas pump, the farmer can't raise the price of his commodity to cover the cost.

The most unpredictable factor is the weather. An unexpected spring blizzard killed thousands of head of cattle on the prairies a couple of years ago, immediately costing those ranchers hundreds of thousands of dollars. When there was drought in the Southwest multiple years in a row, ranchers ran out of feed for cattle and had no way to get it to them without paying extremely high transportation costs. A number of ranches closed their doors and, consequently, cattle numbers went down, pushing beef prices higher in the grocery store.

WE'RE DOING THE BEST WE CAN WHILE ADAPTING AND EVOLVING

One farmer's response to my research on "what if agriculture is wrong" was "I don't think we're wrong, but we're not always right. We're doing the best we can while adapting and evolving to feed and sustain the world. When we know better, we do better adapting and evolving to feed and sustain the world."

Growing food and getting it to your grocery cart is a complex system. It is one that deserves thoughtful discussion—and recognition of the many layers of profit between what is received at the farm and ranch versus what you pay in the grocery, deli, or restaurant.

As you select food for your family, know there is a farmer or rancher at the start of the food cycle risking a million dollars and their family's heritage while pouring their heart, hard work, and hours into growing food for you.

Table 10   Deli and Foodservice Food Truths

Food Myth	Food Truth
Industrial farming makes my food unsafe.	**Food Truth 11: Food safety starts on the farm and ends in your kitchen.** Proper protocol, including hand washing and transparency in the sourcing of products, is essential in deli and foodservices. Food safety ends in your mouth in this case.
Sound bites and diets promoted by celebrities just make sense.	**Food Truth 24: The media isn't the best source of information about food.** People with firsthand experience and expertise are the best sources for farming and nutrition information, not sensationalized marketing misinformation.
It's unnatural to mess with genetics in plants or animals.	**Food Truth 10: Genes are the coolest ingredient on your plate.** Seedless grapes, better bacon, and higher-protein ice cream are a direct result of understanding—and improving—genetics.
Farmers and ranchers grow food because they're subsidized.	**Food Truth 7: Food costs are a shared concern.** Farming and ranching is a high-risk business with increasing challenges, costs from higher regulations, and expenses.

45

Checkout with Truth, Not Fear or Guilt

FOOD SHAMING

"Who has time for this?" was what I heard from nearly every grocery buyer I talked with.

"What if someone sees me and judges me because of what's in my cart?" asked some.

"I feel like I need a science degree to buy food," others commented.

So how is a mom or dad supposed to know if they're doing the right thing for their family?

Confusion and emotionalism have made food a battleground. The marketing is getting bigger. The misinformation grows. Activists continue to bully. Celebrities and politicians take opinion-based positions instead of looking at the facts. Food shaming persists. As a result of all of this, food buyers are filled with guilt and confusion and/or are overwhelmed.

I feel your pain. Unless I have a child along to try to teach them about making healthy choices, my grocery trips are known for speed—grab and go. Be done with it. Partially because I have the patience of a gnat, but mostly because I understand the system behind the food. I know the people raising food are doing it the right way for the right reasons. There are thousands of farmers just like those who have shared what they do throughout this book. I also believe USDA, FDA, and EPA protocols protect our food. I know the science involved and trust it.

> **Food Truth**
>
> Buying and eating the right food doesn't have to be time consuming.

But every issue addressed in this book hits me when I go to the grocery store. I can't just grab a bag of potatoes, pick up a steak, or select cereal without thinking about the people and practices it took to produce that food. That's when the misleading claims about farm families and today's farming and ranching practices become personal.

WHAT ARE YOUR FAMILY'S ETHICAL, HEALTH, ENVIRONMENTAL, AND SOCIAL STANDARDS?

Stick to those and measure all food claims accordingly. The truth in food lies in the way it was produced, how you choose it, and the value it brings to your family. That is ultimately YOUR decision, and you don't need approval from an outside party. My hope is that this book has armed you with the truths so you, too, can ask better questions and adjust as necessary.

I also know people just want to feel good about their food choices. Hopefully this book armed you with truths about food so you can feel good that you are doing the right thing as you buy, enjoy, and serve food.

Apply the food truths on the next trip to the grocery store. Print a wallet copy of the 25 Food Truths from www.causematters.com. Leave it in your kitchen to refer back to when a question or debate comes up.

My mantra is to know the farmer, know the science, or know the system.

In other words, do you have firsthand perspective on how food is raised and why a farmer or rancher uses certain practices? Or, do you know the science behind the food claims to check that it's common sense? Or do you know the agricultural and food regulatory system well enough to trust it?

WANT TO SAVE TIME AND HASSLE AT THE STORE?

Here are three quick ways you can cut down on the clutter and confusion when buying food.

1. Go back to the basics. If a claim causes you to question it and say "wait a minute," it is likely sensationalized and you should walk away.
2. Know your family's ethical, health, environmental, and social standards—and measure all food claims against those.
3. If you know farming, science, or the food system, you can stay focused on buying food that is right for your family—and quickly cut through the claims.

Michele's Food Philosophy

THE FINAL WORDS

When it comes time for my obituary to be written, I hope my legacy will include, "A woman who loved deeply and lived fully. A mom who tried her best. A person who served a calling to connect the worlds of farm and food. She cared about getting back to the truth in food—raised the right way by the right people for the right reasons."

One of my driving beliefs is food is central to a family's well-being. "Dinner is ready!" is the most-mentioned phrase when I have asked audiences for their favorite food quote. I believe that's because it evokes memories of family meals and happiness around food. Let's get back to joy in food.

I WROTE THIS BOOK BECAUSE I CARE ABOUT HONORING THE TRUTH—BOTH FOR YOUR FAMILY AND MINE

My aim in this book was to lift the veil on today's farming and ranching practices—helping you eliminate confusion and bring clarity to your grocery cart.

In my research, many people asked how I personally make decisions in the grocery store, so here's my food philosophy—a baker's dozen on buying and eating food, in case it's helpful to you.

1. Choice matters, both on the plate and on the farm.
2. The circle of life includes dirt, bacteria, genes, DNA, and chemicals. Move on.

3. Size doesn't define the farm or ranch. Family does.
4. Everything in moderation. Including chocolate. And Cheetos.
5. Practice critical thinking; evaluate content and context before drawing conclusions.
6. Measure all food claims against your ethical, healthy, environmental, and social standards—without righteousness.
7. Trust the Nutritional Facts Panel and ignore label marketing claims; there's nothing wrong with nonorganic foods and store brands.
8. Calories in, calories out. If you consume them, take the responsibility to burn them off.
9. Innovation in food production has far-reaching benefits in food, nutrition, medicine, health, and environmental stewardship. Learning why is worth it.
10. Nutritional advice needs to be from a certified registered dietitian making science-based recommendations, not an uncertified nutritionist selling a product, a celebrity promoting a food fad, or a self-made online food diva with no scientific credentials.
11. Likewise, land and animal care perspective needs to be from a farmer or rancher, not an organization with a financial incentive.
12. Variety is essential—on the food plate and in how food is raised.
13. Hungry people around the world deserve quality food resulting from modern-day farming practices.

LEAVE THE GUILT AT HOME AND GIVE YOURSELF PERMISSION TO BE SMART ABOUT FOOD

The truth in food lies in the way it was produced, how you choose it, and the value it brings to your family. Find the truth from the people with firsthand involvement. Use the truth to help your family. Talk about the truth to empower others. The more people who understand and discuss about truth in food helps all of us.

When possible, speak the truth about food and don't allow marketing misinformation to go unchecked. Keep this book handy to use in future food conversations. Go to my site and print out a wallet-sized list of food truths or get a refrigerator magnet to remind you of the 25 truths. You will always be eating, and this issue is not going away—it's going to evolve. I hope this material will serve as an ongoing resource to help you make choices when buying, preparing, serving, and eating food.

Try the 25 food truths the next time you go to the grocery store or have a conversation around food—remember food is designed to bring people together. **Enjoy food as a celebration!**

A Note About the Remaining Aisles and Issues . . .

In this book, I did not discuss each of the 42,000 products you'll find in the grocery store, nor did I touch on every issue and aisle. It's simply too vast of a field to adequately cover in one book.

As I was writing, I realized I'm never going to be able to answer every question, so I focused on those asked the most.

Eating is a deeply personal choice, as is farming. There are a variety of opinions about what is right. Stop and question food marketing claims. Recognize misinformation and why food is produced the way it is by farm and ranch families. Take this framework of 25 truths to shop and eat without guilt.

Keep asking questions and connect with me (@mpaynspeaker) if you want more information.

This is not the end of a conversation, just the beginning.

Notes

2. ARE HAPPY COWS ON DRUGS HARMING MY KIDS?

1. Juskevich, J., and C. Guyer. "Bovine Growth Hormone: Human Food Safety Evaluation." *Science* 249, no. 4971 (1990): 875–84. doi:10.1126/science.2203142.

2. Burckhardt, Peter, Bess Dawson-Hughes, and Connie Weaver. *Nutritional Influences on Bone Health*. Dordrecht: Springer, 2010.

3. Bales, Raymond R., and C.W. Bauman. "Recombinant Bovine Somatotropin (rbST): A Safety Assessment." July 14, 2009. http://www.naiaonline.org/uploads/White Papers/RecombinantSomatotropinASafetyAssessment2010.pdf.

4. Kaplowitz, Paul. "Pubertal Development in Girls: Secular Trends." *Current Opinion in Obstetrics and Gynecology* 18, no. 5 (2006): 487–91. doi:10.1097/01.gco.00002 42949.02373.09.

5. Pape-Zambito, D.A., R.F. Roberts, and R.S. Kensinger. "Estrone and 17β-estradiol Concentrations in Pasteurized-homogenized Milk and Commercial Dairy Products." *Journal of Dairy Science* 93, no. 6 (June 2010): 2533–540. doi:10.3168/jds.2009-2947.

6. "Chapter 2 Shifts Needed to Align with Healthy Eating Patterns." A Closer Look at Current Intakes and Recommended Shifts. Accessed January 28, 2016. http://health .gov/dietaryguidelines/2015/guidelines/chapter-2/a-closer-look-at-current-intakes-and -recommended-shifts.

7. "Questions and Answers about Labeling of Milk Products Containing Recombinant Bovine Somatotropin (rbST)." FoodInsight.org. Accessed October 20, 2015. http:// www.foodinsight.org/Questions_and_Answers_About_Labeling_of_Milk_Products _Containing_Recombinant_Bovine_Somatotropin_rbST_

3. YOUR MILK IS NOT FILLED WITH ANTIBIOTICS

8. USA. FDA. U.S. Department of Health and Human Services Public Health Service Food and Drug Administration. *Grade "A" Pasteurized P Milk M Ordinance O.* 2009 Revision.

9. "Toddler—Food and Feeding, Evidence." *American Academy of Pediatrics*. Accessed September 8, 2016. https://www.aap.org/en-us/advocacy-and-policy/aap-health-initiatives /HALF-Implementation-Guide/Age-Specific-Content/Pages/Toddler-Food-and-Feeding .aspx.

10. "Vitamin D Deficiency in Kids." *The Academy of Nutrition and Dietetics*. Accessed September 8, 2016 http://www.eatright.org/resource/food/vitamins-and-supplements /nutrient-rich-foods/vitamin-d-deficiency-in-kids.

4. ANIMAL WELFARE IS 24-HOUR CARE

11. "Pets or Pensions?" *Humane Watch*. May 18, 2011. http://www.humanewatch .org/pets_or_pensions.

12. Dillard, John. "The Myth of the Humane Society of the United States." *University of Richmond School of Law Juris Publici*. January 2010. http://www.nwsams.com/themyth/.

6. IS ORGANIC THE UTOPIA?

13. "Organic Standards." *United States Department of Agriculture*. September 8, 2016. https://www.ams.usda.gov/grades-standards/organic-standards.

14. "Organic 101: Understanding the "Made with Organic"*** Label." *United States Department of Agriculture*. December 2, 2016. http://blogs.usda.gov/tag/gmo/.

15. Miller, Henry I. "The USDA 'Organic' Label Misleads and Rips Off Consumers." *Forbes*. March 7, 2016. http://www.forbes.com/sites/henrymiller/2016/03/07/the-usda -organic-label-misleads-and-rips-off-consumers/#5067e226536a.

16. Whoriskey, Peter. "Your Favorite Organic Brand Is Actually Owned by a Multi-national Food Company." *Washington Post*, May 6, 2015. https://www.washingtonpost .com/news/wonk/wp/2015/05/06/your-favorite-organic-brand-is-actually-owned-by-a -multinational-food-company.

8. PECKING ORDER ISN'T PRETTY

17. "CSES Research Project." Coalition for Sustainable Egg Supply. Accessed September 8, 2016. http://www2.sustainableeggcoalition.org/research.

9. EGGSTRAVAGANZA OR OVERWHELMED?

18. "When and Why Was FDA Formed?" U.S. Food and Drug Administration. Accessed November 4, 2015. http://www.fda.gov/AboutFDA/Transparency/Basics/ucm214403.htm.

19. "About USDA—A Quick Reference Guide." March, 2016. http://www.usda .gov/documents/about-usda-quick-reference-guide.pdf.

20. Henneman, Alice, and Joyce Jensen. "Cracking the Date Code on Egg Cartons." Accessed January 17, 2016. http://food.unl.edu/cracking-date-code-egg-cartons.

10. FARMERS BUY FOOD, TOO

21. "Survey: Americans Prioritize Affordability and Nutrition over Non-GMO, Organic and Antibiotic-Free Foods." The Chicago Council on Global Affairs. October 14,

2015. https://www.thechicagocouncil.org/press-release/survey-americans-prioritize-aff ordability-and-nutrition-over-non-gmo-organic-and

22. "Bird Flu Pushes Egg Prices to Record Highs, USDA Says." August 12, 2015. http://www.ibj.com/articles/54427-bird-flu-pushes-egg-prices-to-record-highs-usda-says

23. Finz, Stacy. "As New Law Kicks In to Be Kinder to Chickens, We're Shelling Out More for a Carton of Eggs." Cal Alumni Association. January 20, 2015. http://alumni .berkeley.edu/california-magazine/just-in/2015-02-10/new-law-kicks-be-kinder-chickens -were-shelling-out-more

24. Ibarburu, Maro. "The California Situation: A Special Report." Egg Industry Center. December 29, 2014. http://www.internationalegg.com/wp-content/uploads/2015/11 /The_California_SituationIEC_Copy01_06_14_1.pdf.

11. IS YOUR FRUIT CREATING AN
ENVIRONMENTAL FRENZY?

25. Reiley, Laura. "Tampa Bay Farmers Markets Are Lacking in Just One Thing: Local Farmers." Tampa Bay, Florida News. April 13, 2016. http://www.tampabay.com/projects /2016/food/farm-to-fable/farmers-markets/.

26. Desrochers, Pierre and Hiroko Shimizu. *The Locavore's Dilemma: In Praise of the 10,000-Mile Diet.* PublicAffairs, 2012.

27. Bailey, Ronald. Editorial reviews. *The Locavore's Dilemma: In Praise of the 10,000-Mile Diet.* Amazon.com. Accessed September 8, 2016 http://www.amazon.com/The -Locavores- Dilemma-Praise-000-mile/dp/1586489402.

28. 2015–2020 Dietary Guidelines. USDA, Choose My Plate, Accessed September 8, 2016. https://www.choosemyplate.gov.

12. WHERE FRUITS GROW, BUGS GO

29. Wolchover, Natalie. "What Are the Ingredients of Life?" LiveScience. February 2, 2011. http://www.livescience.com/32983-what-are-ingredients-life.html.

30. "Natural vs. Man-Made Chemicals—Dispelling Misconceptions." Compound Interest. 2014. Accessed December 17, 2015. http://www.compoundchem.com/2014/05 /19/natural-vs-man-made-chemicals-dispelling-misconceptions.

31. Industry Statistics: An Overview of the U.S. Apple Industry. Accessed October 25, 2015. http://www.usapple.org/index.php?option=com_content&view=article&id =179&Itemid=285.

32. Postharvest Information Network. "Ethylene: The Ripening Hormone." Accessed March/April 2016. http://postharvest.tfrec.wsu.edu/pages/PC2000F.

13. EXCUSE ME, THERE'S A CUCUMBER IN MY PAPAYA

33. "Hawaii Papayas | Hawaii Grown Papaya." Accessed September 23, 2015. http:// www.hawaiipapaya.com/#gmo-papayas.

34. "Biotech Goes Local: GM Papaya in Hawaii." Biotech in Focus. November 2014. http://www.ctahr.hawaii.edu/biotechinfocus/images/bulletinpdf/Bulletin_Issue21.pdf.

35. "Transgenic Virus Resistant Papaya: From Hope to Reality for Controlling Papaya Ringspot Virus in Hawaii." Accessed September 23, 2015. http://www.apsnet.org/publi cations/apsnetfeatures/Pages/papayaringspot.aspx.

36. "Spittin' Seeds? Not with Seedless Watermelons." Best Food Facts. June 19, 2015. http://www.bestfoodfacts.org/food-for-thought/seedless-watermelons.

37. "How'd We 'Make' a Nonbrowning Apple?" Arctic Apples RSS2. 2011. Accessed September 9, 2016. http://www.arcticapples.com/how-did-we-make-nonbrowning-apple.

38. "Frequently Asked Questions on Genetically Modified Foods." World Health Organization. Accessed September 9, 2016. http://www.who.int/foodsafety/areas_work/food-technology/faq-genetically-modified-food/en.

39. "Over 80 Percent of Americans Support Mandatory Labels on Foods Containing DNA." *Washington Post*. January 17, 2015. https://www.washingtonpost.com/news/volokh-conspiracy/wp/2015/01/17/over-80-percent-of-americans-support-mandatory-labels-on-foods-containing-dna/.

14. CUTTING BOARDS AND CROSS-CONTAMINATION

40. LaGrange Loving, Anna and John Perz. "Microbial Flora on Restaurant Beverage Lemon Slices." Features. Accessed January/February 2016. http://www.pccc.edu/uploads/Xu/1x/Xu1xPvHvoXeYex8Gf1Uh0Q/JEH_Dec_07_with_Copyright.pdf.

41. "Bacteria—Dictionary Definition." Vocabulary.com. Accessed October 16, 2015. https://www.vocabulary.com/dictionary/bacteria.

42. "FDA Taking Closer Look at 'Antibacterial' Soap." December 16, 2013. http://www.fda.gov/forconsumers/consumerupdates/ucm378393.htm.

15. ORGANIC PRODUCE REQUIRES PESTICIDES?

43. "How Wrong Is the Latest 'Dirty Dozen List'?" Biology Fortified, Inc. May 19, 2013. http://www.biofortified.org/2013/05/dirty-dozen/.

44. "Foods Known to Contain Naturally Occurring Formaldehyde." Accessed December 6, 2015. http://www.cfs.gov.hk/english/whatsnew/whatsnew_fa/files/formaldehyde.pdf.

45. "Frequently Asked Questions." April 6, 2011. https://www.americanchemistry.com/ProductsTechnology/Formaldehyde/Answers-to-FAQs-about-the-Health-Effects-of-Formaldehyde.PDF.

46. "History of Bt." Accessed March 2016. http://www.bt.ucsd.edu/bt_history.html.

47. Nester, Eugene, Linda S. Thomashow, Matthew Metz, and Milton Gordon. "100 Years of Bacillus Thuringiensis: A Critical Scientific Assessment, 2002." ASM Academy. 2002. Accessed December 8, 2015. http://academy.asm.org/index.php/food-microbiology/417-100-years-of-bacillus-thuringiensis-a-critical-scientific-assessment.

48. "Organic Production and Handling Standards." USDA Organic. Accessed November 14, 2015. https://www.ams.usda.gov/sites/default/files/media/Organic Production-Handling Standards.pdf.

49. "ECFR—Code of Federal Regulations." Accessed December 4, 2016. http://www.ecfr.gov/cgi-bin/text-idx?SID=43bfede4ca85cda31c8ab17ca8e47da6&mc=true&node=sg7.3.205.g.sg0&rgn=div7.

50. "Organic versus Conventional Foods: Is There a Nutritional Difference?" Best Food Facts. July, 31, 2015. http://www.bestfoodfacts.org/food-for-thought/nutritional-difference-organic.

17. DOES EATING HEALTHY COST MORE?

51. "USDA ERS - U.S. Agricultural Trade: Import Share of Consumption." Accessed February/March 2016. http://www.ers.usda.gov/topics/international-markets-trade/us-agric ultural-trade/import-share-of-consumption.aspx.

52. "Today's Dietitian." Accessed January 5, 2016. http://viewer.zmags.com/publication /1b2da3ad#/1b2da3ad/.

18. VEGETABLES MAKE CHEMICALS?

53. "Natural Toxins in Food." Food and Safety Information Council. Accessed April 20, 2016. http://foodsafety.asn.au/natural-toxins-in-food/.

19. FRESHNESS IS A SCIENCE

54. "A Fresher Vegetable." Morning Ag Clips. February 11, 2016. https://www .morningagclips.com/a-fresher-vegetable/.

20. WHAT'S GROWING IN YOUR VEGGIE DRAWER?

55. Buzby, Jean C., Jeffrey Hyman, Hayden Stewart, and Hodan F. Wells. "The Value of Retail- and Consumer-Level Fruit and Vegetable Losses in the United States." *Journal of Consumer Affairs* 45, no. 3 (2011): 492–515. doi:10.1111/j.1745-6606.2011.01214.x.

56. "USDA and EPA Join with Private Sector, Charitable Organizations to Set Nation's First Food Waste Reduction Goals." USDA News Release #0257.15. September 16, 2015. http://www.usda.gov/wps/portal/usda/usdahome?contentid=2015/09/0257.xml&navid =NEWS_RELEASE&navtype=RT&parentnav=LATEST_RELEASES&edeployment _action=retrievecontent.

57. "Wasted Opportunities: Food Waste Problems and Solutions." *The Huffington Post.* January 12, 2015. http://www.huffingtonpost.com/damon-corywatson/wasted-oppor tunities-food_b_6452420.html.

23. ARE ANTIBIOTICS AWFUL?

58. Hurd, Scott. "No Need to Worry About Antibiotic Residues in Meat." August 15, 2013. http://beta.nationalhogfarmer.com/health/no-need-worry-about-antibiotic-residues -meat?utm_test=redirect&utm_referrer=https%3A%2F%2Fwww.google.com%2F.

59. Waksman, Selman A. "What Is an Antibiotic or an Antibiotic Substance?" *Myco-logia* 39, no. 5 (1947): 565–569. doi: 10.2307/3755196.

60. "Residue Detection Program." Dispositions/Food Safety: Residue Detection Pro-gram. April 11, 2015. http://www.fsis.usda.gov/wps/wcm/connect/ea169f59-0b40-4c77 -8fe1-f04fb00da9e6/PHVt-Residue_Detection_Program.pdf?MOD=AJPERES.

61. "Antibiotics and Animals Raised for Food: Lies, Damn Lies and Statistics." *Food Safety News.* January 7, 2013. http://www.foodsafetynews.com/2013/01/antibiotics-and -animals-raised-for-food-lies-damn-lies-and-statistics/#.V9LGavkrKUk.

62. "IMS Health Study Identifies $200+ Billion Annual Opportunity from Using Medicines More Responsibly." IMS Heath. June 19, 2013. http://www.imshealth.com/en

/about-us/news/ims-health-study-identifies-$200-billion-annual-opportunity-from-using
-medicines-more-responsibly.

63. Raymond, Richard. "Antibiotics and Animals Raised for Food: Lies, Damn Lies and Statistics." Food Safety News. January 7, 2013. http://www.foodsafetynews.com/2013/01 /antibiotics-and-animals-raised-for-food-lies-damn-lies-and-statistics/#.Vs4JKZMrJ24.

64. U.S. Food and Drug Administration. "Fact Sheet: Veterinary Feed Directive Final Rule and Next Steps." December 17, 2015. http://www.fda.gov/AnimalVeterinary /DevelopmentApprovalProcess/ucm449019.htm.

65. Barber, David A. "New Perspectives on Transmission of Foodborne Pathogens and Antimicrobial Resistance." *Journal of the Academy of Nutrition and Dietetics* 218, no. 10 (May 15, 2001): 1559–1561. http://avmajournals.avma.org/doi/abs/10.2460/javma.2001.218.1559.

24. IS MEAT MESSING WITH YOUR HORMONES?

66. Loy, Dan. "Understanding Hormone Use in Beef Cattle." Iowa Beef Center. March 2011. http://www.iowabeefcenter.org/information/IBC48.pdf.

67. Ibid.

68. Ibid.

69. "Chapter 2 Shifts Needed to Align with Healthy Eating Patterns." A Closer Look at Current Intakes and Recommended Shifts. Accessed February 19, 2016. http://health .gov/dietaryguidelines/2015/guidelines/chapter-2/a-closer-look-at-current-intakes-and -recommended-shifts.

70. Bruner, Ann B., Alain Joffe, Anne K. Duggan, James F. Casella, and Jason Brandt. "Randomised Study of Cognitive Effects of Iron Supplementation in Non-anemic Iron-deficient Adolescent Girls." *The Lancet* 348, no. 9033 (1996): 992–996. doi: 10.1016/ s0140-6736(96)02341-0.

71. Rodriguez, N.R. "Introduction to Protein Summit 2.0: Continued Exploration of the Impact of High-Quality Protein on Optimal Health." *American Journal of Clinical Nutrition* 101, no. 6 (2015). doi:10.3945/ajcn.114.083980.

25. THE MASS PRODUCTION OF EDUCATION, MEDICATION, AND FOOD

72. Johnston, Gene. "PEDV Dominates the Pig World." September 11, 2014. http:// www.agriculture.com/livestock/hogs/health/pedv-dominates-pig-wld_284-ar45068.

26. DOES YOUR BURGER DAMAGE THE ENVIRONMENT?

73. "Sources of Greenhouse Gas Emissions." U.S. Environmental Protection Agency. Accessed September 12, 2016. https://www.epa.gov/ghgemissions/sources-greenhouse-gas -emissions.

74. "Beef's Shrinking Footprint." International Animal Law. December 23, 2011. http://www.animal-law.biz/node/653.

75. Bailey, Arthur W. "Management of Canadian Prairie Rangeland. Ottawa: Agriculture and Agri-Food Canada, 2010." http://www.beefresearch.ca/files/pdf/fact-sheets /991_2010_02_TB_RangeMgmnt_E_WEB_2_.pdf.

76. "Is Feedlot Beef Bad for the Environment?" *Wall Street Journal*. July 12, 2015. http://www.wsj.com/articles/is-feedlot-beef-bad-for-the-environment-1436757037.

77. "Turkey Farmer—A Sustainable Entrepreneur in Michigan." Cause Matters Corp. 2010. http://www.causematters.com/articles/turkey-farmer-thanksgiving/.

27. THERE IS NO SINGULAR "RIGHT" WAY TO BUY OR GROW FOOD

78. Kelly, Jerry. "Dynamics of the Meat Case." North American Meat Institute. February 21, 2016. http://www.meatconference.com/sites/default/files/books/Jerry%20 Kelly%20-%20Dynamics%20of%20the%20Meat%20Case.pdf.

79. "Animal Production Claims Outline of Current Process." September, 2016. http://www.fsis.usda.gov/wps/wcm/connect/6fe3cd56-6809-4239-b7a2-bccb82a30588 /RaisingClaims.pdf?MOD=AJPERES.

28. ARE YOU GROWING BACTERIA?

80. Friedman, Lindsay. "The Art of Hand Washing Has Yet to Be Mastered." *USA Today*. June 22, 2013. http://www.usatoday.com/story/news/health/2013/06/22/hand-wash/2438613/.

81. Salter, Jim. "Hospitals Seek High-Tech Help for Hand Hygiene." *USA Today*. June 28, 2013. http://www.usatoday.com/story/news/nation/2013/06/28/hospitals-techn ology-hand-hygiene/2471443/.

29. SAVING OUR SOIL

82. "Five Fascinating Facts About Soil." CropLife International. December 4, 2014. https://croplife.org/news/five-fascinating-facts-about-soil/.

83. Hogg, John, and Melvin D. Joesten. *Chem 2: Chemistry in Your World*, 2nd ed. Boston: Cengage Learning, 2015.

30. WOULD YOU LIKE A LOAF OF GUILT WITH YOUR BREAD?

84. Jones, Julie. "Wheat Belly—An Analysis of Selected Statements and Basic Theses from the Book." Cereal Foods World (July/August 2012). http://www.aaccnet.org/publi cations/plexus/cfw/pastissues/2012/OpenDocuments/CFW-57-4-0177.pdf.

85. Kasarda, Donald D. "Can an Increase in Celiac Disease Be Attributed to an Increase in the Gluten Content of Wheat as a Consequence of Wheat Breeding?" *Journal of Agricultural and Food Chemistry*. January 11, 2013. http://pubs.acs.org/doi/abs/10.1021/jf305122s.

86. Miller Jones, Julie. "Are New Wheat Varieties Really Making Us Fat and Sick?" March 19, 2016. https://chs.asu.edu/sites/default/files/jones.pdf.

31. SUGAR, SALT, AND EVERYTHING EVIL

87. Sollid, Kris. "Sugar: Not So 'Simple' Anymore." FoodInsight.org. August 15, 2014. http://www.foodinsight.org/NotSoSimpleSugar.

88. Espat, Adelina. "Does Cancer Love Sugar?" MD Anderson Cancer Center. May 2015. https://www.mdanderson.org/publications/focused-on-health/may-2015/FOH-cancer-love-sugar.html.

89. "Sugar 101." American Heart Association. Accessed September 12, 2016. http://www.heart.org/HEARTORG/HealthyLiving/HealthyEating/Nutrition/Sugar-101_UCM_306024_Article.jsp#.V9crrfkrKCg.

90. Zelman, Kathleen. "Iodine, a Critically Important Nutrient." www.eatright.org. November 3, 2015. http://www.eatright.org/resource/food/vitamins-and-supplements/types-of-vitamins-and-nutrients/iodine-a-critically-important-nutrient.

91. "Executive Summary." Office of Disease Prevention and Health Promotion. Accessed September 9, 2016. https://health.gov/dietaryguidelines/2015/guidelines/executive-summary.

32. IS YOUR FAT BETTER THAN MY FAT?

92. Kuzemchak, Sally. "The Truth About Saturated Fats." *Fitness magazine.* September 2012. http://www.fitnessmagazine.com/recipes/healthy-eating/nutrition/good-and-bad-fats/.

93. "Amount, Types of Fat We Eat Affect Health and Risk of Disease." Accessed December 4, 2016. http://www.todaysdietitian.com/news/012914_news.shtml.

94. "Nutrients and Health Benefits." Choose MyPlate. May 20, 2016. http://www.choosemyplate.gov/nutrients-and-health-benefits#sthash.6K4xJjI3.dpuf.

34. THE DEMONIZATION OF THE CORN STALK

95. "Fast Facts about High-Fructose Corn Syrup." Accessed November 2015. http://www.foodinsight.org/Content/3862/HFCS FACT SHEET - FINAL.pdf.

96. "Corn Refiners Counter Sue the Sugar Association." September 4, 2012. http://corn.org/corn-refiners-counter-sue-the-sugar-association.

97. Fitch, Cindy, and Kathryn S, Keim. "Position of the Academy of Nutrition and Dietetics: Use of Nutritive and Nonnutritive Sweeteners." *Journal of the Academy of Nutrition and Dietetics* 112, no. 5 (May 2012): 739–758. Accessed November 2015. http://www.andjrnl.org/article/S2212-2672(12)00325-5/pdf.

35. IS THE ENVIRONMENT SACRIFICED FOR PROFITABILITY?

98. "Banning GMOs Would Negatively Impact Environment, Economies." *Corn and Soybean Digest.* March 1, 2016. http://m.cornandsoybeandigest.com/issues/banning-gmos-would-negatively-impact-environment-economies?NL=SO-02RESP.

99. Savage, Steven. "Why I Don't Buy Organic, and Why You Might Not Want to Either." *Forbes.* March 19, 2016. http://www.forbes.com/sites/stevensavage/2016/03/19/why-i-dont-buy-organic-and-why-you-might-want-to-either/#535121c11c2e.

100. "Historical Farm Data Reports." MnSCU Farm Business Management Annual Report. 2014. http://fbm.mnscu.edu/annualreports/2014/fbm_s456_2014_annual_report.pdf.

101. Ibid.

36. WHAT IS PECKSNIFFERY?

102. "Monthly Storm Water Tips." DarbyBorough.com. May 2016. http://darbyborough.com/wp-content/uploads/2010/01/May-2016.pdf.

37. THE REALITY OF CONVENIENCE

103. Clayton, Joseph. "Celebrate National Frozen Food Month!" FoodInsight.org. March 10, 2016. http://www.foodinsight.org/frozen-food-month-packaged-foods-myplate-nutrition-pizza-fruits-vegetables-meals.

40. ARE THEY SNEAKY SNACKS OR ARE WE LABEL ILLITERATE?

104. Mikkelson, David. "Dangers of Dihydrogen Monoxide." Snopes. Accessed February 23, 2016. http://www.snopes.com/science/dhmo.asp.

105. Jesper, Emily. "Making Sense of Food Additives." Sense About Science. Accessed April 21, 2016. http://www.senseaboutscience.org/data/files/resources/121/Making-Sense-of-Food-Additives-v8.pdf.

106. U.S. Food and Drug Administration. "Overview of Food Ingredients, Additives & Colors." November 2004. http://www.fda.gov/Food/IngredientsPackagingLabeling/Food AdditivesIngredients/ucm094211.htm#qalabel.

41. WHOSE HANDS HAVE BEEN IN YOUR FOOD?

107. "Hand Hygiene Statistics." Minnesota Dept. of Health. Accessed April 24, 2016. http://www.health.state.mn.us/handhygiene/stats/.

108. Doheny, Kathleen. "Most Common Foods for Foodborne Illness: CDC Report." Medscape. January 30, 2013. http://www.medscape.com/viewarticle/778455.

109. Raymond, Matt, and Laura Kubitz. "IFIC Foundation Research Highlights Changes in Consumers' Perceptions of Food Safety Risks." FoodInsight.org. September 1, 2015. http://www.foodinsight.org/press-releases/ific-foundation-research-highlights-changes-consumersâ€™-perceptions-food-safety-risks.

110. Beach, Coral. "Massachusetts Chipotle Closes Because of Norovirus." Food Safety News. March 8, 2016. http://www.foodsafetynews.com/2016/03/massachusetts-chipotle-closes-because-of-norovirus/#.VxqwVJMrJGN.

42. JUST BECAUSE YOU CAN'T PRONOUNCE IT DOESN'T MEAN IT'S BAD FOR YOU

111. Spector, Dina. "What It Would Look Like If Your Banana Came with an Ingredient List." Business Insider. January 20, 2014. http://www.businessinsider.com/ingredient-list-for-natural-products-2014-1.

112. "Monocultures—the Great Evil of Modern Ag?" Thoughtscapism. March 17, 2016. https://thoughtscapism.com/2016/03/17/monocultures-the-great-evil-of-modern-ag/.

113. "WHO Clarifies IARC Report Linking Red, Processed Meat to Cancer." The International Center of Excellence in Food Risk Communication. October 30, 2015. http://www.foodriskcommunications.org/content/who-clarifies-iarc-report-linking-red -processed-meat-cancer.

43. WE'RE NOT CROSSING FROGS AND CORN

114. Senapthy, Kavin. "Girl Scouts' Science-Based GMO Stance Worth Cookies' Dollar Price Increase." *Forbes*. November 12, 2015. http://www.forbes.com/sites/kavinsenapathy /2015/11/12/girl-scouts-science-based-stance-worth-dollar-price-increase/#398f63242a3e.

115. "FAQs: Girl Scout Cookies." Girl Scouts of the USA. Accessed March 22, 2016. http://www.girlscouts.org/en/cookies/all-about-cookies/FAQs.html.

116. Keller, Rich. "Greenpeace Only Has Scare Tactics against GMOs." The Sensible Environmentalist. June 25, 2012. http://www.ecosense.me/index.php/views-articles/8-views /15-issues-6.

117. "FAQ's on Genetically Modified Foods." World Health Organization. Accessed April 4, 2016. http://www.who.int/foodsafety/areas_work/food-technology/faq-genetically -modified-food/en/.

118. Kyndt, Tina, Dora Quispe, Hong Zhai, Robert Jarret, Marc Ghislain, Qingchang Liu, Godelieve Gheysen, and Jan F. Kreuze. "The Genome of Cultivated Sweet Potato Contains Agrobacterium T-DNAs with Expressed Genes: An Example of a Naturally Transgenic Food Crop." *Proceedings of the National Academy of Sciences* 112, no. 18 (March 2015): 5844–5849. doi:10.1073/pnas.1419685112.

44. EVERYTHING IN MODERATION

119. Rodenburg, Jack. "Robotic Milking Gets More Affordable Every Year." Time for Technology. Accessed April 23, 2016. http://www.dairylogix.com/15- Robotic Milking is getting more affordable every year.pdf.

Index

About the Author

MICHELE PAYN brings clarity and common sense to the grocery store. Known as one of North America's leading farm and food connectors, she is passionate about getting back to the truth in food—raised the right way, by the right people, for the right reasons.

Payn is an in-demand media resource whose work has appeared in USA *Today*, *NPR, CNN, Food Insight, Food & Nutrition Magazine, Grist, Technorati*, and others. Michele has spoken for hundreds of groups, including dietetic associations, universities, Genome Prairie, Michigan Vegetable Growers, the Farm Credit Council, the Apple Processors Association, and farm bureaus in 30+ states.

In addition to nearly 40 years of firsthand farm experience, she has:

- Authored *No More Food Fights! Growing a Productive Farm & Food Conversation*, a book presenting opposing views to help people around the food plate connect at the center through civilized conversation.
- Founded AgChat and FoodChat, virtual communities connecting more than 20,000 farmers, dietitians, chefs, foodies, agribusinesses, and ranchers from 20 countries since 2009, now managed by a not-for-profit she helped create, the AgChat Foundation.
- Earned the Certified Speaking Professional designation awarded to less than ten percent of professional speakers globally, after speaking for 500+ groups.
- Received BS degrees in Animal Science and Agricultural Communications from Michigan State University, where the story of her impact has been featured in a *Spartan Saga*.
- Worked with farmers in 25 countries, raised millions of dollars for education, and built a successful business, Cause Matters Corp.

Michele Payn is a mom who enjoys working on her small farm in Indiana with her daughter.

Connect with @mpaynspeaker across social media:

- Twitter: http://www.twitter.com/mpaynspeaker
- Facebook: http://facebook.com/causematters
- Instagram: http://www.instagram.com/mpaynspeaker
- LinkedIn: https://www.linkedin.com/in/mpaynspeaker

Have these food truths helped you shop and eat with less guilt? Do you have food truths you'd like to explore? Are questions popping up as you buy food with a new awareness? Michele would love to hear from you; you can email book@ causematters.com.

Want to arrange for Michele Payn to translate farm to food for your conference, company, or organization? Discover yourself why audiences rave about Michele's high energy, interactive programs, and unique ability to engage everyone around the table. Learn more about her speaking and training programs at www.causematters.com.